20,000 SECRETS OF TEA

An ancient Chinese proverb says:
Better to be deprived of food for three days
than of tea for one.

Tea has been a favorite beverage worldwide for hundreds of years. A cup of tea on a rainy evening can chase the chills away and a pot of tea shared among friends can lend an air of enchantment to an afternoon. But more than that, tea can treat a variety of ailments, and with this invaluable guide you can put the secrets of tea to work for you!

- Sage tea in the middle of the afternoon will make you feel like your day is just beginning.
- Peppermint tea eases pain, headaches, and is a general cure-all.
- Rosemary tea on your scalp can help to stimulate hair growth.
- Thyme tea, considered the most powerful antiseptic herb, helps to heal infections, infectious diseases, and septic conditions.
- Chamomile in your bath will totally relax you and do wonders for your skin.

And much, much more!

20,000
Secrets of
❧ TEA ❧

The Most Effective Ways to Benefit from Nature's Healing Herbs

Victoria Zak

A DELL BOOK

Published by Dell Publishing
a division of Random House, Inc.
New York, New York

Dell books may be purchased for business or promotional use or for
special sales. For information please write to: Special Markets
Department, Random House, Inc., 1540 Broadway,
New York, N.Y. 10036.

ISBN: 978-0-440-23529-3

Printed in the United States of America

Published simultaneously in Canada

Designed by Kathryn Parise

November 1999

20 19 18 17 16 15 14 13

OPM

This book is dedicated to Leona.

Acknowledgments

First, I'd like to say a heartfelt thank-you to my agent, Sally McMillan. I'd also like to thank my editor, Christine Zika; editorial assistant Caroline Sincerbeaux; and photographer Alexa Garbarino and associate art director Marietta Anastassatos for their superb cover design. Special thanks for support to Donald Axinn, Shannon Banks, Stacey Chase, Tina D'Amato, Charles Facey, Rose Fidel, Tasha and Steve Halpert, Pat Klinzing, Claire Lehrman, Joan Mason-Quigley, Judith Podell, Cris Carlin Scheidt and Phil Scheidt, Sylvia Stickney, Peter Vash, Judy and Cliff Wagner, and Kathy Zak. I'd also like to thank all the herbalists and herbal gardeners who have kept the tradition of herbs alive throughout the generations.

"When I drink tea
I am conscious of peace
The cool breath of Heaven
rises in my sleeves, and
blows my cares away"

——CHINESE POET LOTUNG

Contents

෨

Foreword

The father of medicine—Hippocrates—was once quoted as saying, "Let your food be your medicine and your medicine be your food." In the following piece of literature, the wisdom of the author reveals the healing properties of natural plants that have been in use for over four thousand years. This book could not have been written in a more timely fashion, as we are now entering an age where illness is reaching epidemic proportions.

Many of the pharmaceutical drugs we have today have their origins in natural plants, and many new medicines will be discovered in our rain forests in the near future. Conventional medicine has saved many lives with its advanced technology, and I know many people who are alive today thanks to a particular type of drug or surgery that is available in our medical arsenal. But I also believe that many more will be saved by knowing the truth about natural plants, so that we can use the plants as God intended: "And the fruit there shall be for meat, and the leaf for medicine." —Ezekiel 47:12.

It is in every person's best interest to learn and know about our planet and the plants that grow on it.

Charles E. Facey, ND,
Doctor of Naturopathy, Master Herbalist, and
Certified Homeopath and Holistic Consultant

Introduction

❧

My own life has been so enriched by herbs and herbal teas that I want to share my enthusiasm with you. Like many people, I've tried herbs in myriad forms, but I can honestly say that I haven't found another way to take herbal remedies for health treatments that can match the simplicity, grace, and effectiveness of herbal teas.

As you venture further into this book to learn more about herbs and herbal teas, I hope you will always remember to use a good measure of common sense for your guide.

A study in 1996 on consumer preferences interviewed people who did not take herbs, asking them if they planned to take herbs in the future. The study revealed that 63 percent of more than one thousand people surveyed plan to take herbal supplements within five years as "the answer to many common ailments" or "part of our daily regimen." Among those surveyed, 60 percent said they would take herbal remedies for energy enhancement, 56 percent said they would take them to prevent colds, 54 percent to boost immunity, and 43 percent to help them sleep. If that population sampling holds on a national scale, it means that more than half of the population could be taking herbs in the near future, which will make herbal remedies even more popular than they are today.

What's the best way to take herbs safely and with confidence? Armed with information. It's essential to know the nature of every substance you put into your body. If you're like most health-conscious consumers today, you don't hesitate to ask your doctor or pharmacist for the available information and potential side effects of prescription medications, and you should be equally as circumspect with herbs.

Keep these commonsense guidelines in mind when you use herbs as health treatments, whether you use them as teas or in other forms.

Herbs shouldn't be used as substitutes for a healthful diet and lifestyle, but as complements to it.

Herbs should never be used as substitutes for a doctor's prescription.

If you are being treated for any illness and are taking prescription medication for that illness, seek your doctor's consent for herbs you might be considering, either alone or as complementary therapies.

Herbs should not be taken by pregnant women, nursing mothers, or children without their doctor's consent.

The renowned medical herbalist Penelope Ody recommends that you do not start taking a "tonic" herb while you are in the throes of an illness. Since tonic herbs can be potent, your best course might be to wait until the illness subsides before adding a tonic herb to your health menu, or seek professional guidance.

Know all about the herb *before* you take it.

It's often been said that health is wealth. When you are well informed about herbs, you have a wealth of knowledge on your side that can save you a lot of time, trouble, and costly mistakes when you are choosing and using herbs. That way, you can add the richness and pleasure of herbs to your daily life and reap true health benefits.

Welcome to the wonderful world of herbal teas. Enjoy!

🙾 1 🙾

The Wonders of Tea

It's been called the plant of Heaven.

For 4,000 years, it's been valued both as a medicine and a drink for pleasure.

Tea

Originally, *tea* referred to one species of shrub that was cultivated in China—*Camellia sinensis*—known as the black tea shrub.

A charming legend tells how this ordinary plant became the first natural wonder in the world of herbal teas.

The story takes us back to ancient China in 2737 B.C. when one day, Emperor Shen Nung was kneeling before a fire, heating water. Suddenly a wind stirred. Leaves fluttered down from a branch over his head and fell into the boiling water. The aroma captivated Shen Nung and he decided to taste the brew.

Where did these aromatic leaves come from? An ancient wild species of the black tea shrub. When the leaves are fermented, they produce oolong or black tea, but when they are brewed fresh, as in Shen Nung's tea, they yield the refreshing green tea, which contains the potent antioxidant *catechin*, a bioflavonoid with antibacterial and anticancer properties.

For centuries in China, monks and herbalists studied plants for their healing properties, and handed down their knowledge to the next generation by verbal instruction. To illustrate the importance of tea, a tale tells of an ancient Chinese herbalist who knew 100,000 healing properties of herbs, and began to pass on his wisdom to his son. The herbalist taught his son 80,000 secrets, but fell ill before he could complete the lessons. On his deathbed, the herbalist told his son to come to his grave five years from the date of his death, and there he would find the other 20,000 secrets.

On the fifth year, the obedient son went to his father's grave, and found, growing on the site, the black tea shrub.

The black tea shrub is a plant that has been endowed with the Taoist belief that beauty and harmony are achieved by order and ritual. Every detail in the planting, picking, preparation of the leaves, and ceremonial customs for drinking tea became a cultural phenomenon in the Orient. It was passed on to other cultures as humble gifts from Buddhist monks. When Japanese monks journeyed to China to study with Chinese monks, they returned home with seedlings from the black tea shrub as parting gifts. Today, Japan specializes in the production of green teas, now known as its national beverage. The plants that grow in Japan today are thought to be offshoots of those first seedlings.

The black tea shrub is a plant that has sailed the world on clipper ships and trade routes. In 1559, a tea merchant from Persia told a Venetian scholar about his experience in China, drinking tea. The scholar wrote an account of the merchant's tea tale that set the port of Venice buzzing. What was this mysterious brew? Everyone wanted to taste it. By the early 1600s, the Dutch East India Trading Company was bringing shipments of dried herbs from the black tea shrub in specially lined boxes to Europe.

Tea was such precious cargo in its early years of import to Europe, it was reserved for royal tables, or tea-tasting parties of the rich and influential. It was introduced as an exotic medicinal beverage that could promote longevity and cure many disorders. The herb's price exceeded one hundred dollars per pound. But the herb wasn't the only expense involved.

To follow the Chinese custom, tea-drinking ceremonies in Europe required imported china. Tiny Ming teacups from China were made of porcelain and held only a few sips of tea. The cups rested on porcelain saucers, and to brew the tea, a proper Chinese teapot was needed, along with a Chinese tea jar to store the dried leaves. This was a costly endeavor that kept tea out of reach for average people. At the time, the process for making porcelain was not known in Europe, and to curb the import costs for drinking tea, the Dutch developed an imitation of the Chinese tea service in elegant blue and white delftware.

One of the earliest tea parties on record in America was held in 1674 in the Dutch Colony of New York (then called New Amsterdam). To taste the newly imported teas, society ladies arrived in their best dresses, carrying their own teacups, fashioned from delicate china, with bowls the size of wineglasses. To this day, many herbalists still specify herbal tea doses as "the size of a small wineglass."

A hundred years later, the Sons of Liberty brewed up the most memorable tea party of them all. In 1773,

Americans had independence on their minds, and Britain's prohibitive taxes on tea sparked a revolution. Thirty-two cases of expensive dried herbs were tossed into the harbor on the night of the Boston Tea Party. It was the signal for the birth of a new nation.

For an ordinary plant, the black tea shrub has quite a few tales to tell of romance and intrigue, old worlds and new worlds, culture and customs. But it wasn't the only plant in the tea garden.

Locally grown herbs had been used for teas all over the world, and traded in their own way, though not as aggressively as black, oolong, and green teas. Many Mediterranean herbs were brought to Europe by the early crusaders and the Roman army. Other herbs followed the trade routes of saffron to the far east, and were exchanged for black tea leaves.

Early American colonists learned the secrets of locally grown herbs from the Indians, and these discoveries played an important role in the fight for independence. To protest the British taxes on tea in 1773, American women in Boston, Hartford, and other New England cities vowed to drink teas from indigenous weeds instead of imported teas. The brews they came up with were called *Liberty Tea*. Among them were the antiviral flowers of chamomile, calcium-rich raspberry leaves, and wild American sage, which is so admired by the Chinese as an herb for longevity that it remains a major American export to China today.

The Universal Garden

Through the ages, as the black tea plant mingled with herbs from many cultures, *tea* took on a broader meaning to encompass a wide variety of herbs, and now refers to a

brew made from the leaves, flowers, berries, seeds, roots,
rhizomes, or bark from a plant, steeped in hot water.

The generic term *plant* acquired the more cultivated
name *herb* in botany, the branch of medical science de-
voted to the study of plants. More than 3,000 herbs have
been studied and catalogued with properties that are
healing to the human system, and not all of the plants
have been studied. Some of our best western drugs were
derived from herbs, including the heart medicine *digitalis*
from the herb foxglove, and the asthma-aid *ephedrine*
from the herb ephedra, and for years, these drugs con-
tained the original herbs as ingredients. It wasn't until
World War II, when herb shortages in Europe limited the
production of these drugs, that scientists persevered by
designing synthetic versions.

Each herb has its own history and folklore that are as
captivating as the tale of the black tea shrub.

Some herbs, like mint, were so valued in biblical
times that they were used to pay taxes. Other herbs were
honored as religious plants and dedicated to gods and
goddesses. The gold flowers of calendula (pot marigold)
are regarded as a remedy to strengthen the heart, and the
herb has been held in high esteem in many religions. In
Greek myth, the creation of calendula was attributed to
Artemis, goddess of the moon, sister of the sun god,
Apollo. In India, Buddhists consider the plant sacred to
the goddess Dwiga, and its flowers adorn her emblem.
Calendula was given many names in many countries, all
associated with *gold*. When Christianity became the pre-
dominant religion in Europe, and many medicinal herbs
were renamed to harmonize with the new religion, calendula was given the name *Mary's Golde* or *Marigold*, in
honor of the Virgin Mary.

Herbs have been found in monastery gardens and
royal gardens all over the world, from ancient times to

the present. If you look closely, you'll see the wound-healer yarrow and the herb of wisdom, sage, growing in the gardens of the National Cathedral in Washington, D.C.

Herbs as Healing Foods

Hippocrates said, "Thy food shall be thy medicine," and herbs, as concentrated foods with vital nutrients, vitamins, and medicinal properties, more than fill the bill. In Hippocrates' time, herbs were the official medicines. Throughout the ages, people in every culture have taken herbs for their healing benefits in the same way we take garlic or eat oranges, for the vital nutrients these herbs provide, and their special restorative value to the human body.

In our current medical climate, we've been fore-warned that synthetic antibiotics are proving to be ineffective against new viruses. Where do we turn to treat common disorders like colds, the flu, skin eruptions, and hosts of low-grade infections that crop up regularly and keep us from feeling our best? If you turn to herbs, you will find that there are more antiviral, antifungal, and antibacterial herbs than you ever dreamed.

More and more scientists are returning to herbs as sources for new medicines. Many modern-day hospitals are including naturopathic clinics as part of their treatment facilities, to provide a wider range of options for care. It's a signal that the new medicine for the millennium will include more natural alternatives for treatment, and a new view of the oldest treatments in the world—herbs.

The World of Herb Teas

Teas are herbal drinks, and because of that, they can do much more than quench your thirst or calm you after a long day. Teas are the ideal way to get the healing power of herbs into your everyday diet. Drugless remedies. Natural energy. Pure and simple drinks that can provide effective herbal defenses against disease.

I'd like to introduce you to the wonderful world of teas. In this book, you'll find more than one hundred herbs for teas with special healing properties. There's power in those flowers, leaves, roots, rhizomes, berries, seeds, and bark—positive plant energy that is absorbed easily and gently through teas.

There are immunity-building teas to strengthen your body's own natural defenses, or to rebuild your strength after antibiotics, illness, or surgery. There are stress reducers, nervous-system soothers, and antianxiety teas. You'll find natural antacids for indigestion, natural antihistamines to fight hay fever and allergies, and natural antidepressants. There are teas to tone specific body systems, "Chi" teas, to enhance vital energy, tonics for both sexes, and teas for your golden age. A pharmacopoeia of herbal teas is at your beck and call.

You can drink your herbal teas as you like them—hot or iced, plain or sweetened. You can prepare them the easy way, from ready-made tea bags, or you can use dried or fresh herbs, and filter the bulk from the liquid before drinking your tea. Whatever way you like them, you'll be amazed at the potential for drugless healing that is available in herbal teas.

Herbal teas are a natural solution for people who want to get the protective health benefits of herbs in their daily diet, but don't feel comfortable taking handfuls of herbs as capsules, and rarely use more than the standard herbs like garlic and basil for cooking.

Herbal teas are a valuable resource for people who don't want to rely on pills for minor discomforts and ills.

In our complicated world, it's nice to know that there are still some plain and simple solutions to make our everyday lives easier.

You'll even find some unexpected uses for herbal teas. Herbal teas are pure herbal waters that can be used as skin washes or on compresses to heal wounds and reduce inflammations, since your skin is also a transmitter for vital nutrients. They can also be herbal remedies for your bath, and when you steam an herb in a pot of boiling water, it's aromatherapy in the air.

Many herbs come in ready-to-use tea bags that are portable for travelers. They take up no space in a suitcase and fit in the back pocket of your tightest jeans. There's even a tea for travelers' blight—dysentery—and that's billberry tea.

Herbal teas have been making people feel better for centuries, and the average person who wasn't a monk, herbalist, or botanist probably had no idea why. They drank teas and felt better, so they drank them again.

Take chamomile tea, for instance. You might drink chamomile for its soothing feeling or as a sleep-aid, without realizing that it also treats irritable bowel syndrome, eases indigestion, and has antibacterial properties to keep infections away. That's a soothing reason to keep drinking chamomile tea. Or peppermint tea. You might like peppermint for its refreshing taste, without realizing you are also treating your liver to a tonic, fighting nasal congestion, and cooling inflamed joints. Or rosemary, the herb of remembrance. That's not just a sentimental adage about rosemary. The tea increases the circulation to your brain, which enhances alertness and memory.

There's a wonderful world of teas to drink for their special benefits.

And when you do, it will be like rediscovering the Garden of Eden in simple, pleasing drinks.

For natural healing, all you have to do is . . .

> steep
> and
> pour.

❧ 2 ❧

Sympathetic Remedies

"Better to be deprived of food for three days than of tea for one."

—ANCIENT CHINESE PROVERB

Herbs are not magic potions reserved for dark rooms, musty shelves, and colored bottles. They're plants that grow in sun or shade; some flower, some bear fruit, some are showy, others are plain, some are woody, and others downy.

In the roots, leaves, flowers, berries, bark, or seeds, herbs have specific biochemical properties that are healing and restorative for our systems. Cranberry, for instance, has naturally occurring calcium. That's good news for people who need calcium and aren't milk drinkers. Dandelion has potassium and is a mild diuretic. That's important news for people who need to prevent fluid retention, but can't afford the potassium losses common to standard diuretics. Dong quai is rich in vitamin E and minerals for a vital energy tonic that can be exceptionally good for menopausal women. Ginseng, an immune system stimulant known as the king of tonics for men, also helps to regulate blood sugar and cholesterol levels.

Herbs do their job because of the properties they contain. There's no magic in it, just biochemistry. We've come to the point in our high-stress lives where we need all of the healing and restoration we can get. Herbs are there to help us.

The Unique Value of Herbs as Teas

Herbal teas are the most effective way to get the benefits of herbs, safely and easily.

UNCOMPROMISED VALUE

Herbal teas are true natural resources! They have no additives, preservatives, or dyes. They aren't sweetened with sugar or sugar substitutes, and they're not mixed with other ingredients that could compromise the herb's effect or give you something you don't want or need. They are also available in caffeine-free varieties.

EASY ABSORPTION

The water in herbal teas plays a vital role to increase the effectiveness of the remedy. Water is essential in your body for the absorption and assimilation of nutrients. The water diffuses the potency of the herb and delivers its properties in a manner that is harmonious with your natural body processes. Unlike herbal capsules that never touch your taste buds, herbal teas follow the normal digestive process from your mouth through your system, which is an automatic regulator for substances entering your body.

Dose Control

Many herbs come in premeasured tea bags that take the guesswork out of measuring herbs. Premeasured tea bags insure that you are taking enough of the herb without taking too much. A standard tea bag contains one teaspoon of a dried herb. One teaspoon is a good measure to use for a remedy—a moderate dose of herbs that is safe and effective. With one teaspoon as a measure, even if you use dried herbs in an infuser to make your herbal tea, you have a standard to use for dose control.

Cutting Through the Confusion

There are hundreds of herbs with healing properties, and each herb has its own unique virtues. As a consumer, you can often be overwhelmed with expensive and varied ways to take herbs—in capsules as a single herb or in blends, as tinctures with alcohol or glycerine, in vials, packets, or premixed formulas. This can become so muddled and costly that the world of herbs becomes a garden of confusion. Herbal teas cut through the confusion about using herbs. They make dealing with herbs a down-to-earth experience.

Years of Tradition

Herbal teas have centuries of tradition to back up their use. They've been used as drinks for pleasure and healing remedies in every culture, throughout the world.

Affordability

Herbal teas are the most cost-effective way to get the benefits of herbs at an affordable price. An average box of tea contains twenty-four tea bags for twenty-four cups of tea, and the average cost is less than five dollars per box. That's about twenty cents per cup. Dried herbs can be purchased from herb shops by the ounce, giving you more versatility in herbal selections and even more savings than you get with ready-made tea bags. Herbs that were once reserved for the tables or medicine shelves of royalty are now affordable and available to everyone!

Teas for Two Reasons—Double Benefits

One of the remarkable qualities about many herbs is the fact that they can do more for your body than merely treat symptoms. In many cases, they can treat the symptoms *and* an underlying weakness.

If you get hay fever, for instance, and take elderberry tea to relieve your stuffiness and congestion, you are deriving other benefits too. While elderberry relieves the symptoms of allergies and hay fever, it also treats an underlying weakness—elderberry strengthens your respiratory tract by helping to remove imbedded phlegm and mucous from the lungs, and it reduces inflammation. A stronger respiratory system is your best defense against allergic reactions in the future.

Many herbs have properties that strengthen particular organs or body systems, and when you use them, you may notice that you derive unexpected benefits as well. Milk thistle contains *silymarin*, a flavonoid that helps to rejuvenate your liver, one of the primary organs for detoxifying your system. When you take milk thistle tea to tone your liver, skin problems can improve, depression can lift, headaches can be less frequent, and you might notice that you have more energy. These problems are often associated with a weak liver, and they can abate as you strengthen the organ that was weak.

When you take herbs as teas, you get the benefits of

the herbs and some delightful drinks too. They add pleasure to your daily menu, and they add a whole new di-
mension to healing.

Where Do You Start?

ONE TEA A DAY IS BETTER THAN NONE

Start very simply, and seek out one herbal tea that
might be useful for your current needs, such as papaya
tea, if you suffer from acid indigestion and routine digestive distress.

More than one hundred herbs are highlighted in this
book, with a brief description of each herb, its folklore,
its uses in history, its properties and values. You'll probably be surprised to see how many vitamins and minerals
you can receive from one cup of herbal tea. Along with
each herb's profile, you'll also find ideas for special teas.

TWO TEAS A DAY ARE BETTER THAN ONE

If you find two herbal teas to help you, that alone
would make your discovery of herbs worthwhile. Over
time, as you learn to trust the gentle relief and healing
benefits that herbal teas bring, you'll find more teas to
help you resolve everyday disorders as they surface.

Then you might want to try a few herbal teas that
have deeper, disease prevention properties. Astragalus is
a splendid tea to try if your immunity has been weak-
ened by too many rounds of antibiotics, recent surgery,
or if you suffer from exhaustion and feel totally depleted
of strength. Oatstraw is a full-body tonic and a natural
antibiotic. Slippery elm is especially good for intestinal
stress, including colitis, and it helps to heal inflamed conditions throughout the body.

Then one day you might notice that you feel calmer and more energetic than you used to feel; you don't seem to get colds as easily as you used to; and when you face those everyday ills, you have some reliable methods for dealing with them.

That day, you'll realize that you've made a breakthrough. You might look at the boxes of tea or collection of dried herbs on your shelf and pause in amazement. Plain and simple drinks. Plain and simple healing.

That's the beauty of herbal teas!

How Much—and How Often—for Health Treatments?

You don't need to take handfuls of herb capsules, or drink the same tea ten times a day to reap the benefits of an herbal remedy. One great tea, once a day, is a positive step forward. Two great teas a day can be a real health advantage.

If you are just starting to use herbs for their healing properties, I would recommend that you begin with moderate doses, like the dose in one cup of tea in the morning. If you struggle with depression or nervous tension, for instance, try St. John's wort tea. You will notice its soothing effect immediately, and the herb will continue to work its way through your system for the next several hours. If you are fighting a tough and recurrent problem with depression and tension, you might try St. John's wort again in the evening. But there's no need to take the tea again in the evening, if one tea in the morning soothed you all day.

When you are using teas for healing treatments, a good rule is to take the tea as you need it, once or twice a day, and use it for one week.

After a week, evaluate your progress. If the problem has abated, there's no reason to take the tea every day.

You can use the tea intermittently, for a tune-up.

The best way to use herbs for healing is to use a moderate approach, since herbs work slowly and steadily to relieve your symptoms and balance your system as well.

One or two cups of an herbal tea, in the morning and evening, is a very successful treatment. Try it! I think you'll agree.

Targeting Your Tea—Starting With Simples

To target your herbal tea, refer to Chapter 5, which provides an **Herbal Guide to Health.** It gives you a list of common health problems and health-oriented needs in A-Z format, followed by a selection of herbal teas that can be used for treatment.

Start With Simples

Identify the herb most suited to your current health needs and buy ready-made tea bags with that herb, or the dried herb to make your tea. A tea made from only one herb is called a *simple*, meaning that the herb is the only ingredient in the tea—nothing is added to sweeten or enhance it, and it is not combined with other herbs.

If you are a newcomer to the garden of herbal teas, and want to use an herb for a specific treatment, like eyebright tea if you suffer from tiredness and eyestrain from too much computer work, your best bet is to buy the *simple*—plain eyebright tea. That will allow you to get the true, rich taste of the herb, as well as allow you to evaluate how you feel while drinking it, and how your system responds to it. It will also give the herb the best chance to do what nature designed it for, with speed and efficiency, because the herb is in its pure state.

Using *simples* for treatments helps you avoid confusion about herbs, and teaches you about each herb as you drink it.

You can find boxes of *simple* teas at your local health food store. Often, health food stores will stock a complete selection of plain herbs for teas, from A-Z—alfalfa to yarrow, or they can order a specific herbal tea for you. The herbs in boxes will come in tea bags or in bulk form (the dried herb). Check the box to insure that you are getting the form you desire—*tea bags* or *bulk*.

Some of the more familiar herbs like chamomile, peppermint, and ginkgo can be found in supermarkets, pharmacies, and grocery stores, but there is one cautionary note. Be sure to check the list of ingredients to be certain that the only constituent is the herb alone. If the list of ingredients says that it uses a "flavoring" instead of an herb, that tea will not necessarily give you the specific benefits you are seeking. For instance, you might want to try raspberry tea for its healing effect on the urinary tract. In a supermarket, you find a tea that is called "Raspberry Tea," but when you read the ingredients, you discover that it contains black tea with raspberry flavoring. While the black tea can be a delightful drink with its own virtues, you are looking for plain raspberry tea made from the herb raspberry.

Teas for Pleasure and Treatment

You can look at the world of teas in two equally pleasant ways:

• *Tea for Pleasure—Health Benefits Extra.* Since there are so many herbal teas with exquisite tastes, you can select your teas for pleasure alone, and get the health benefits as a bonus.

For instance, sage has a woodsy, brisk, and spirited taste, and it has antioxidants to prevent premature aging of cells. Rosemary is piney, fragrant, and tender to the taste, and it's also a circulatory tonic that helps to digest fats. Fenugreek has a deep, nutty flavor and it's comforting for stomach disorders. Chinese oolong, which helps to lower cholesterol levels, has been called light, rich, lush, and refreshing, reminiscent of an herb garden after a summer shower.

• *Tea for Treatment.* If you take an herbal tea for its specific health properties, the best way to take it is *plain*. That way, you will get to know your healing herb as well as any expert can, by personal taste, and personal response, and you have a world of herbal teas to choose from. When you feel run-down and can't seem to find your old energy, or if you struggle with lingering disorders, then the plainest-tasting teas can become your favorites, because they work so well.

When I first started my discovery of herbal teas, I took the teas plain and couldn't believe the surprising tastes of many of the less common herbs. Some charmed me the minute they touched my lips, while others seemed bland, boring, or even mildly bitter at the first taste. But a funny thing happened to me. Since I was taking an herb tea for a particular health benefit, I suspended my judgment on the first taste, in favor of the effect. In just about every case, the effect was better than I dreamed, so I continued to drink the particular herbal tea, regardless of the taste. Over time, I found that some tastes I thought I disliked at first were now intriguing. I began to long for the taste of bitter brews, because they were so good to me. My internal response was to crave what was healing. Herbs with bitters are excellent regulators for the digestive system, and now I'd say the taste of an herb tea with bitters is something to savor like a fine, aged wine.

A friend of mine had a similar experience. She used to prefer teas with honey, or sweetened tea blends, because she likes sweet foods and drinks. Then one day, she caught an intense head cold and wanted to put it in check as quickly as she could. She suffers from allergies and bouts of asthma, so in her case any infection in her sinuses can lead to more serious consequences. In her frustration with the cold, she was less concerned with taste and more interested in results. She took plantain tea *plain*, an herb with an all-business taste and the remarkable ability to pull the toxins out of your mucous linings and dry a head cold fast.

The next day, she called and said her head started clearing within twenty minutes after taking the plantain tea, so she shut off her phone and went to bed. With former colds, because of her asthmatic condition, she often wound up in the hospital for a night, because she has a difficult time with many over-the-counter cold medications.

Since then, she's been taking herbal teas plain, some with tastes that would have seemed unusual to her before, and she loves them without sweeteners. She also claims that when she drinks the herbal teas with bitters, she craves less sugar. That's another benefit of bitters in herbs, they stabilize your digestion.

Many herbalists say that you should get to know an herb you are taking, and in a sense, develop a friendship with it, learn to admire its taste and virtues. That way, healing works better.

Bags or Bulk Tea

READY-TO-USE TEA BAGS

Perfect herbal tea is quick and easy with premeasured
tea bags. All you have to do is boil water, pour it in your
favorite cup, drop the tea bag in, and wait 3–5 minutes.
Don't forget to press the potency from the tea bag before
removing it from your cup.

Drink your tea warm, or pour the brew into a tall glass
filled with ice. If you're concerned about the potency of
an herb in tall glasses of iced teas then let your tea steep
longer in hot water to get a stronger brew. Add additional
cold water to fill the glass as needed. Another option is to
make two bags for a full-flavored iced tea. Hot or cold,
good health was never so easy!

BULK HERBS FOR TEAS

Herbs may come as loose dried herbs (bulk) in tea
boxes, or you can buy them by the ounce from herb
shops. Preparing a tea from bulk herbs is easier than you
think. After a while, you'll learn to love this method
because you can make your brew exactly the way you
like it.

To make an ideal tea from bulk herbs without any
extra equipment, put a heaping tablespoon of bulk herbs
into your favorite cup. Boil water in a nonmetal teapot, if
possible. Pour the hot water into the cup, cover the cup,
and let your herbs steep for 3–5 minutes. Strain the bulk
before drinking. That's all there is to it! If you don't
have a teapot to boil water, don't forgo the tea. Use a
saucepan to boil the water, nonmetal if possible.

To strain your tea, you can use a nylon sieve, a small
strainer, or—if you have none of these accoutrements

available—you can use an unbleached coffee filter. It's better than skipping the tea.

A great way to make bulk teas is to use a tea infuser, available at your supermarket or health food store.

Spoon Infuser. A spoon-sized metal infuser opens to fit your dried herbs inside, and closes to put in your tea cup. It has holes on the sides of the spoon to release the properties into the water, without the bulk. Purists might argue that it's not the best choice, because it's metal.

Strainer Infuser. A circular plastic spoon infuser has strainers on both sides to allow the brew to be made without bulk in the water. It fits a heaping tablespoon of dried herbs and snaps tightly to enclose the herbs. I found mine at the supermarket in a rack next to the teas.

Tea balls. Tea balls are also available in your health food store or market. It's a small, egg-shaped infuser, with holes in the sides, and a chain, to float herbs right in your teapot, and capture the essence of the herb without the bulk in the water. To use the tea ball, wait until the water in your teapot is briskly boiling, turn off the flame, wait a minute until the water comes off the boil, and insert your tea ball with the bulk herbs inside.

Steep your tea a little longer if you want a richer brew—from five to seven minutes, or up to ten minutes for real strength of character.

You don't need expensive equipment to make a great tea from dried herbs. Remember how the first tea was brewed? Shen Nung's tea was made with leaves that fell into his pot of boiling water under an open fire.

You can make extra tea and store it in the refrigerator to drink later. It will retain its flavor for two days. With teas, color is no indication of strength. Some of the palest tea waters can be the most potent.

Fresh-from-the-Garden Herbal Teas

The taste of an herbal tea made from fresh herbs is exhilarating. And if the herb comes from your own garden, it gives you a sense of satisfaction that is unbeatable. Peppermint, for instance, is so aromatic that you get invigorated with a snap of a leaf. Plant peppermint in your garden to have iced peppermint tea on a hot August day. Freeze the herb fresh, or dry it for future use, to have warm peppermint tea in winter.

You can make your teas from fresh garden herbs, but keep these precautions in mind:

- Never pick herbs in the wilds to use for teas, since you cannot know whether the area was sprayed with chemical insecticides.
- Make sure a neighboring plant isn't woven into the herb you are picking, since plants tend to be friendly with each other.
- Be sure to use the correct parts of the plant for your tea. Each herb has specific parts that are used for their healing properties. For instance, calendula tea only uses the flower petals, but rosemary tea uses the whole plant above the root. To find out which parts of an herb are used, look up the herb you want to pick for your tea, and check the *Beneficent Parts* for that herb.
- Pick the freshest herbs you can get, and wash them thoroughly. Peppermint castile soap is an excellent wash for herbs.

INFUSION METHOD

This method is used for softer parts of a plant, such as flowers, stems, or leaves. Cut your herb into small pieces and use two tablespoons of fresh herb per cup. Pour freshly boiled water over the herb in your cup. Cover the cup and let it stand for 7–10 minutes. Strain and drink.

CONCOCTION METHOD

For fresh tea from the harder parts of a plant, such as bark, twigs, seeds, roots, or rhizomes, a stronger method is needed. Cut the hard parts into small pieces, and measure two tablespoons of fresh herb per cup. Place the herb in a saucepan, cover it with cold water, and bring the water to a boil. Reduce the heat and simmer for one hour. Strain and drink. Extra tea can be refrigerated.

Ginger After Dinner

Pick up a ginger root at your grocery store and try the concoction method to turn it into a fresh ginger-root tea to have as an after-dinner treat. It warms you all over and makes digesting your meal a breeze.

No time? Use a premeasured tea bag of ginger root. Good digestion was never so easy.

To Sweeten or Not to Sweeten

In eastern countries, like China and Japan, *plain* is still considered the best way to take your tea, especially for healing!

In Salem, Massachusetts, purists still take the strongest brews plain.

In Russia, a slice of lemon is the only garnish.

Try your herb tea unsweetened first. Wait to see how it feels in your system. If you aren't comfortable with the plain taste, add a teaspoon of honey to sweeten it.

After you take your tea with honey for a few days, try it once again without honey. If you now like the tea plain, leave out the honey and drink.

Try to resist refined sugar and artificial sweeteners. If you are taking herbal teas as healing remedies, refined sugar or artificial sweeteners diminish your potential for healing. One of the favorite environments for bacteria is sugar. While honey has natural sugar, it also has antibacterial values of its own, and many healthful properties to add to the tea.

In colonial America, teas were topped off with saffron or linden blossoms to charm the brew. You can use:

A hint of mint
A slice of lemon or lime
A squeeze of orange
A stick of cinnamon
A dash of natural vanilla
A touch of sweet anise

LONG LIFE GARNISH

In the Chinese tradition, to wish a guest a long life, dried chrysanthemum blossoms are floated in the cup of tea. That's what I'd wish for you as you begin or renew your adventure into the world of herbal teas.

❧ 3 ❧

The Bounty of Blends

One tea a day is better than none
Two teas a day are better than one

The beauty in a cup of blended tea is the extra boost of healing that an additional herb can bring.

You can add rose hips to echinacea for a cold remedy with extra vitamin C and antioxidant power. You can add peppermint to green tea for aromatic menthol in a vital energy tea. You can add a berry herb to marshmallow for an antiaging tea with a "very berry" flavor.

Blends provide a way for you to individualize your herbal teas. You can create flavors that are richer than the original brew, aromas that elevate your mood as you sip your tea, and you can create synergy—a combination of flavor and energy that literally sparkles with health benefits.

You can make a plain tea tantalizing, a bitter tea sweet, a tart tea mellow, and you can tame a tonic tea to flow gently through your system like a quiet river.

As you get to know the healing virtues in the variety of herbs that are used for teas, you'll probably find that you prefer some herbs over others for their unique tastes or the special benefits you feel when you drink your tea.

You might find that you love the taste of cranberry, but also want the healing benefits of a plainer-tasting tea like milk thistle. That's where blends come in. They provide a means for you to create herbal teas that are inspired by your own tastes and desires, and suited to your particular health needs. You can express your individuality in your blends. You can name your teas and develop blends for special friends. The inspiration that herbs can bring to your life is truly limitless!

Inspirational Blends

You can develop your own inspirational blends with ease. The key is to use *equal parts* of each herb in one cup of tea.

The standard dose for a cup of herbal tea is one tea-spoonful of dried herbs, whether you are using one herb or several herbs.

If you are making a blend with dried herbs, simply divide the herbs into equal parts to total one spoonful.

If you are making a blend with tea bags, which already contain one teaspoonful of an herb in each bag, simply consider each tea bag as a cup of water that you need to add to your blend to account for the higher dose of herbs. For instance, a blend with two tea bags would require two cups of water, while a blend with four tea bags would require four cups of water.

There's no reason you can't combine a tea bag and dried herbs in the same blend, adding more water to account for the increased potency of the tea bag. I do it all the time when I want to make a particular blend and can't find one of the herbs I need in a ready-made tea bag.

A charming feature about blends is the unique nature of people and the individuality they bring to their blends. To give you some examples of the versatility of people, I've sought out some recipes for blends from friends. You can use the recipes to try at home, or you can use them as inspiration to begin to create your own blends.

KATHY'S COLOR HARMONY

Kathy is a watercolorist who sees her blends from an aesthetic perspective, in the same way she sees the merging colors of sunsets, trees, and stones on the paths in her paintings. She selects her herbs for their healing value, and creates blends for their richness of color. She uses different colors for different seasons, and while she's drinking the blend, the color is her inspiration.

Red and purple blends for winter—Kathy uses berry teas like cranberry, raspberry, and blackberry to color winter blends. These are herbs that are rich in minerals and vitamin C to fight colds and flu, and keep her body tuned throughout the cold months. They combine radiantly with plain-tasting herbs.

Bright green and yellow blends for summer and spring—Her selections are light, cleansing herbs like dandelion, parsley, and peppermint which make fabulous iced teas. They're packed with nutrition and give her system a fresh, clean feeling to breeze through spring and summer with renewed energy. They harmonize with each other or brighten a plain brew.

Deep green and amber blends for fall—Her choices are the woodsy teas like plantain, rosemary, and sage, with cinnamon as a garnish. The inner bark of cinnamon is a marvelous infection fighter, and one cinnamon stick is the equivalent of one herb in a blend. Add a cinnamon stick to an amber brew and you get what Kathy describes as "aromatic topaz."

These are some of Kathy's Inspirational Blends:

Iced Peppermint Twist—for instant refreshment, a rush of menthol, great circulation, and health. Equal parts of peppermint and lemon balm, with a spiral orange twist cut from the orange skin to float on the top of a tall glass of iced tea.

Iced Cranberry Dandy—a wonderful internal cleanser and source of nutrition. Equal parts of cranberry and dandelion in a tall glass with ice.

Coco-Roco Red—for chocolate lovers, a rich, tantalizing taste, lots of vitamins and minerals, toning for your organs. One package of cocoa powder (sweetened or unsweetened) and one tea bag of red raspberry.

In the Pink Drink—a fabulous tea to boost your immunity and flood your cells with vitamin C. It's also an excellent cleanser for your urinary tract. Especially nice iced. Equal parts of echinacea and cranberry.

TASHA'S PEACE GARDEN

Tasha is an herbalist, folk singer, and poet, with a lush herb garden that she landscaped in a spiral design. At the beginning of the spiral, there are rows of echinacea, and as the path circles in, new herbs grow at each bend. At the center of Tasha's garden is a still pool of water in a stone shell. She calls it "The Peace Garden," and uses the herbs to make her blends.

A refrain that always stayed in Tasha's mind was "Parsley, sage, rosemary, and thyme," from an old English folk song. As an herbalist, she couldn't resist turning it into a blend.

These are some of Tasha's tried and true blends:

Scarborough Fair Tea—for recovery, clear thinking, and feelings of well-being. It's an uplifting blend that literally sings. Equal parts of parsley, sage, rosemary, and thyme.

Razzle Dazzle—for toning the organs, digestive complaints, and constipation. Equal parts of parsley, raspberry, and basil.

Peace Garden Tea—for cleansing energy and a celebration of life. It's a blend with a calming, refreshing nature, like a walk through an herb garden after a spring rain. Equal parts of lavender, lemon grass, and parsley.

TINA'S TEA TREASURY

Tina is a medical student with a degree in Naturopathy. She'll be a versatile doctor, licensed in both western and herbal medicine. She provided a top-notch health hint when we were talking about blends. Tina likes elder and casually said: "You know, elder is good for anything that ends in *itis*." I responded: "Sinusitis, Colitis, Arthritis, any *itis*?" Tina nodded yes and said, "*Itis* means it's *inflamed*." That makes elder an ideal choice for any blend that is designed to fight inflammation.

These are some of Tina's blends for special treatments:

Allergy Blend (Gentle)—it's antiviral, antiinflammatory, and a decongestant. Equal parts of mullein and elder.

Allergies, Colds, Bronchitis (Vigorous)—a blend with everything for your upper respiratory tract, but it's also fabulous for your overall health. Equal parts of mullein, thyme, marshmallow, elder, and peppermint.

Midafternoon Blahs—a blend for health and aromatherapy. Green tea is a tonic, peppermint stimulates your senses, and lemon grass gives your thyroid a boost. Equal parts of green, peppermint, and lemon grass.

CHARLIE'S ENERGY BLENDS

Charlie is a master herbalist who holds certificates as a Doctor of Naturopathy and Homeopathy, and he owns a country health store. Every day, he's consulted about herbs to take for modern-day concerns and he knows what's hot. He advocates using common sense and calls his remedies "Common Sense Blends."

Energy for Men—for vitality and anti-aging, body and brain. Equal parts of Siberian ginseng and gotu kola.

Energy for Women—for hormone balance, flow of "Chi" energy, and harmony. Equal parts of dong quai and chaste berry.

Prostate Tune-up—to cleanse and strengthen the reproductive organs. Equal parts of saw palmetto and rose hips.

Blood Pressure Stability—a sweet, warming blend to help to prevent buildup of plaque on arterial walls, break down fats, and improve circulation to the extremities. This, in turn, helps to stabilize blood pressure and improve the heart's functions. Equal parts of flax and ginger.

CLAIRE'S SPIRIT OF NATURE

Claire is a mother, herbalist, and artist. She has a generous nature and love for herbs that makes an average conversation like a course in botany.

This is Claire's whole-health blend:

Digestive Tonic—a synergistic blend that eases stomach discomfort, tones the digestive tract, lifts your spirits, and heightens energy. Rich, aromatic brew. Equal parts of raspberry, licorice, and peppermint.

Herbs to Use for Your Blends

Flavor and Synergy. Following the tradition of the great teas, there are some tried-and-true herbs that have been added to blends for flavor and synergy for centuries. They are:

1. Any of the lemons—lemon balm, lemongrass, lemon verbena
2. The primary mints—peppermint and spearmint
3. The sweetest herbs—licorice and anise
4. Floral herbs (they are also aromatic)—hibiscus, linden blossoms, chamomile
5. Fruits and berries—raspberry, blackberry, elderberry, rose hips.

These standards often appear as routine features in ready-made blends. They are often used for flavor, but since they are herbs that bring virtues of their own to a blend, they also create synergy.

To make a little magic with your own blends, rely on the lemons, mints, sweets, florals, fruits, and berries for flavor and synergy.

Five Tastes

In Chinese medicine, taste is an important consideration in a prescription for an herbal remedy. Five tastes are linked to different body systems and specific emotions.

Sour—liver, gallbladder, eyes, tendons (and the emotion *anger*). To generate health in these areas, you might try herbs with sour tastes like lemon balm, lemon verbena, lemongrass, or wild strawberry in your blend.

Salty—kidneys, bladder, ears, hair, bones (and the the emotion *fear*). For a health boost in these areas, try salty herbs like plantain, bladderwrack, or cleavers as part of your blend.

Pungent—lungs, large intestines, nose, skin (and the emotion *grief*). To stimulate health in these areas, you might try pungent herbs like sage, hyssop, basil, or ginger as part of your blend.

Sweet—spleen, stomach, mouth, muscles (and the emotion *worry*). To increase vitality in these areas, you might add sweet herbs to your blend, like licorice, rose hips, flax, ginseng, or dong quai.

Bitter—heart, blood vessels, small intestine, tongue (and the emotion *joy*). If you're feeling joyless and tired, you might try a bitter herb like scullcap, lavender, chamomile, or mildly bitter marigold.

One herb has all five tastes—schizandra. You can use it in a blend for balance and harmony.

Ready-Made Blends

There are many premeasured blends of herbal teas that can be found in health stores, convenience stores, country stores, supermarkets, and pharmacies. These blends can contain from one to ten herbs, and sometimes even more.

How Can You Evaluate If a Ready-Made Blend Is Right for You?

A good general rule to follow: the simpler the blend, the easier it is to research the ingredients.

It's essential to know the nature of each herb in a blend before you buy. A few minutes of research can make a big difference in the remedy you choose. It helps you make an informed choice, and makes it less likely that you'll find something you don't like about the blend after you break open the box and steep your first cup. It will save you money, since you won't have "half-tried" treatments stacked on the back of your shelves.

It's also the best policy to look up the herb yourself,

rather than rely on information provided by over-the-counter salespeople. Every person is different, and an herb that might appeal to one individual might not please another. For instance, one person might be comfortable taking the herb ma huang in a blend for energy even though there are cautions that it raises the heart rate, but you might not be as casual about herbs as that person. When you research an herb for yourself, you will be left with no doubts about your selection. Best of all, a few minutes of research can help you single out the blend that will work best for you, then all you have to do is steep, pour, and drink, for immediate relief.

To make that research easier, I've included the profiles of more than one hundred herbs in **A Modern Herbal Tea Garden.** You can look up each herb to discover it's nature and make your decision armed with information. If you can't find an herb in my collection of profiles, ask the salesperson to look it up for you. They usually have books behind the counter for their own use. If they can't find the herb in one of their volumes, choose another blend. There are so many wonderful, wholesome herbs to choose from, you don't need to take a risk on a "mystery" herb.

1. Simple Blends With One-to-Five Herbs. Many simple blends with one-to-five herbs have been standards for years and have provided people with pleasant-tasting teas for common disorders such as colds, flu, sleeplessness, PMS, arthritis, and rheumatism. New breeds of simple blends are appearing every year, with modern desires in mind—energy, vitality, antiaging, immunity, and relief from digestive disorders, anxiety, and depression.

As a rule, simple blends rely on tried-and-true herbs that will appeal to the greatest number of people and have the most wholesome ingredients. One or two herbs in the blend will be the primary healing ingredients, with

additional herbs added to enhance the flavor and synergy, to make the tea pleasing to the greatest number of
people. The flavor and synergy herbs are the five standards mentioned in more detail earlier—*lemons, mints,
sweets, flowers, fruits, and berries.* These standards are often
found in blends for a wide range of disorders, so you'll
only have to look them up once to cover the bases for a
variety of blends.

When it comes to primary herbs in simple blends,
some common themes might catch your eye. For instance, chamomile seems to be a standard in blends for
sleeping; echinacea is often found in blends for colds and
flu; and ginseng is common in blends for energy. Even
when modern blends contain less familiar herbs, you will
usually find the old standbys as part of the blend. For
instance, a modern sleeping blend may contain valerian
or skullcap, but it will usually contain chamomile as well.

What does this tell you? The standards are the most
reliable, most trustworthy, and the wholesome herbs for
the most people. When in doubt, choose a blend that
uses the standards, and you will be making a selection
that has centuries of tradition to back up its use.

2. Complex Blends With Five-to-Ten Herbs. A
simple technique you can use to evaluate these blends is
count the number of herbs that are used for flavor and
synergy—*lemons, mints, sweets, flowers, fruits, and berries*—
then see what's left over. Look up the herbs that are left
over. Many complex blends are really simple blends with
a greater number of lemons, mints, sweets, flowers,
fruits, and berries. If the majority of the herbs in a complex blend are unknown to you, and don't use the standards for flavor and synergy, consider that blend a
"complicated blend."

3. Complicated Blends With Ten-or-More Herbs.
Complicated blends are a specialty that should be over-
seen by qualified professionals. If a blend contains ten or

more herbs that are unfamiliar to you, but you trust that particular company's products, look up each one of the herbs, or call the company for information, and make your best judgment call.

If you are just getting acquainted with herbal blends for healing, over-the-counter complicated blends are not the best first choice. There are two drawbacks to consider with complicated blends. I call the problem, *Which Herb Is It?*

Something Doesn't Agree With You. If you take a treatment with multiple herbs in a blend, and one of the herbs doesn't please you or agree with you, there's no way to know *which herb is it?* That could lead you to believe that herbs in general don't work for you, and leave you feeling frustrated about using herbal remedies for relief.

Something Works, But What? If you take a treatment with multiple herbs in a blend, and one of the herbs brings a little relief, there's no way to know *which herb is it?* That leaves you in the dark about which herbs work best for you.

When the number of herbs increases in a blend, the dose of each herb is reduced. In ready-made blends, the standard dose for the entire tea is still one teaspoonful (level or rounded). If there are sixteen herbs in a blend, the dose of each herb has to be divided into sixteen pieces (not necessarily equal parts). The synergy of multiple herbs can maximize the overall effect when it is developed properly, but when it is developed too generally, too many herbs can dilute the remedy.

For the best domestic use, the simpler blends—the ones with fewer herbs—will be your best teachers, and they can be the best healers.

Time-Honored Blends

In the days before modern medicine, herbs as foods and teas were the only treatments people had to fight illnesses and infections.

Families grew their own herbs, or, in many countries, such as England, local parish gardens grew herbs for use by the community. In the early days of medicine, monastic and churchyard gardens were literally the pharmacies for everyday people, and because of that tradition, some of the rarest herbs still survive today.

The panoramic herbal gardens of rulers and kings were designed for beauty, aromatherapy, symbolism, and status, but they were also practical, since the plants provided the pharmaceutical ingredients for royal use.

I've singled out some simple blends that you can try at home with two ready-made tea bags, dried herbs, or a combination of both.

Most time-honored blends are gentle but effective treatments that have proven themselves over and over again through the centuries. Who knows, you may find one old-timer that is precisely the one you need. That's what makes herbal traditions so enriching!

That Wicked Spirit Influenza—for the flu, drink it warm if you have the chills, drink it cool if you feel feverish. Equal parts of elder and peppermint.

A Woman's "Complaint"—for hormone balance and tension relief during PMS. Equal parts of chaste berry and skullcap. If you add a dash of vanilla, it will lift your spirits.

To Sleep Perchance to Dream (Gentle)—to ease tension, anxiety, and restlessness before bed. Equal parts of chamomile and hops. You can sweeten it with honey, which also has sedative properties.

Alas! Sweet Melancholy (Depression)—to strengthen the nerves and chase the cloud of sadness away. Equal parts of chamomile and scullcap. Or equal parts of chamomile and vervain.

The Breath That Seizeth (Bronchial Asthma)—for immediate relief, a bronchial dilator, cleansing and invigorating. Drink it as a hot tea. Equal parts of butcher's broom and green.

That Dastardly Lead (Lead Poisoning)—in the event of an emergency when no doctor is near, this works as a diuretic and cleanser that helps to remove toxins and provides vitamins and minerals for repair. Equal parts of dandelion and rose hips.

Thank You, Mother Nature

There's a hidden benefit in your exploration of herbs that you might find enriching. It can make you look at the world of plants in a whole new way. One day, you might be walking along a road and you'll spot yarrow growing wild. You'll look at its feathery leaves and know they can break a fever if you use them in a tea.

A few blocks up the street, you might see the regal cones of echinacea radiating in the sun. You'll know that the root of that beautiful flower can strengthen your immunity.

Growing in your own backyard, or in the parking lot if you live in an apartment, you'll most likely see plantain, because that herb seems to grow everywhere it's needed to detoxify the soil. You'll know its leaves will detoxify your blood in an emergency.

It makes you feel connected to the land, the greens, the flowers, and the earth because you are learning their secrets.

The world is a garden to enjoy!

Getting to know the herbs can bring a new view of nature to your life. It can make you wide-eyed and wondrous as a kid. That's the beauty of herbs. They're positively inspirational.

4

Teas and Specialties

It took centuries for green and black teas to make their way to Europe from the mainland of China, and another few centuries of export for them to become world-favorite beverages. But with the invention of the tea bag, it only took a "New York minute" to change the tea trade forever.

In the early 1900s, tea merchants shipped their tea samples to potential customers in specially designed tea tins. But New York tea merchant Thomas Sullivan thought the cost of the tins was inflating the price of his teas and hindering their sale. He decided it was cheaper and easier to send tea samples to his customers in small silk bags!

Orders poured in to Thomas Sullivan's office for—of all things—tea in bags!

Later, silk gave way to filter paper, and tea became a more economical drink, affordable to everyone.

Daytime, Nighttime, and Good-Time Teas

There are times of the day when teas pick you up. There are times of the day when teas calm you down.

Any time you use them, herbal teas add their healing value to your life. For an extra health boost, garnish your teas with orange, lemon, or cinnamon sticks and sweeten them with honey or natural vanilla.

Bright and Early Teas—an invigorating way to start your day—try eyebright, green, oatstraw with orange

Midmorning Boost—to keep you going until lunch, and help to curb your appetite—try ginseng, pau d'arco, suma with cinnamon

Luncheon Treats—Light, refreshing teas for a break in the routine—try raspberry, strawberry, peppermint iced

Midafternoon Lift—Teas to make you feel like your day is just beginning—try yerba mate, ginkgo, dong quai

Evening Meals—Teas for accompaniment for meat, fish, casseroles, salad—try rosemary, sage, anise

Quiet Moments—Teas to calm restlessness and ease you into sleep—try chamomile, hops, licorice

The Innovation—Iced Tea

The invention of iced tea was a boon to the tea trade. The event happened in America, but the credit belongs to the British, with a little help from India and Ceylon, who provided the teas.

In the St. Louis World's Fair in 1904, tea merchants from around the world displayed their samples and provided freshly brewed tea for tasting. A representative from India and Ceylon Teas was there, an Englishman from Calcutta named Richard Blechynden.

The crowd was sweating in the St. Louis heat. They

didn't want tea. They wanted cold drinks. Blechynden was a man who could think on his feet. He took tall glasses, filled them with ice, and poured the hot tea over the ice. Eureka! A new cold drink. The crowds went wild for it.

Today, almost half the teas people drink each year are iced teas, and they continue to gain popularity.

True Fruit Iced Teas

Instead of sugary sodas, try true fruit iced teas. You'll get natural energy with more staying power. By drinking true fruit teas instead of sodas, you are reducing the sugar content in your system, which helps you fight infections, since bacteria thrive in sugar. And sip by sip, you are replacing that sugar with herbal nutrition and healing properties.

You can depend on true fruit iced teas for a cool boost of energy and nutrition any time of day.

True Fruit Cranberry. A pretty pink drink, cranberry tea is a renowned healer for the kidneys, bladder, and urinary tract. It keeps E. coli from clinging to bladder walls to prevent infections. Rich in iron and calcium, it also has vitamins A, B-complex, C; citric and malic acids; and minerals.

True Fruit Bilberry. A rich, red drink, bilberry tea helps to preserve vision, protects from eyestrain, and is good for night blindness. It was taken as a jelly by Royal Air Force pilots for night missions in World War II. It helps to lower blood sugar levels, has iron, phosphorus, potassium, manganese, zinc, and fruit acids.

True Fruit Raspberry. This deep amber brew is excellent for your gums and throat. It tones the lower body organs, strengthens the kidneys and urinary tract. It has vitamins A, B-complex, C, E; citric and malic acids; calcium; niacin; iron; magnesium; pectin; potassium; selenium; silicon; sodium; and zinc.

True Fruit Wild Strawberry. The tea with a tint of scarlet and a delicate flavor, wild strawberry is a body tonic with iron to build blood. It's a real energizer and cleanser with citric acids; pectin; vitamins B, C, E; and minerals.

True Fruit Hawthorn Berry. A symbol for hope and joy in Greece, hawthorn berry is a heart tonic and circulatory stimulant. It improves oxygen uptake, which helps to regulate heart rate and stabilize blood pressure. It's abundant in nutrients, including vitamins C, A, B-complex; silicon; iron; selenium; and potassium.

True Fruit Rose Hips. A vibrant amber-red brew, rose hips tea is a true healer for everything from skin hydration to the cells of your innermost being. It's an antiaging tonic and aphrodisiac with lots of vitamins and minerals to fight fatigue and give you vitality. It's especially nice iced.

Herbal Ice for Special Occasion Teas

A fresh sprig of mint in each ice cube before you freeze them is a charming way to give your guests a mint treat in their iced tea. You can also make ice cubes with tea, and add the extra herbal flavor to your drink right in the ice cube. Try lemon balm ice cubes for flavor and synergy in any tea.

Simplify Slimming With Teas

Herbal teas provide a natural way to help you lose excess weight.

Weight problems are exacerbated by digestive difficulties, stress, and poor circulation which hinders the assimilation of nutrients and elimination of wastes. Herbal teas with bitters ease digestive disorders, cleanse your body, and bring new vitality to your system. Herbal teas that are diuretics help to prevent water retention and bloating. Some herbal teas strengthen your resistance to stress, so you automatically lose the cue for stress-eating.

Herbal teas have no calories or fat. There are sweet teas to ease sugar cravings and teas to aid in the digestion of carbohydrates, proteins, and fats. You never have to feel depleted of energy with the vitamins, minerals, and nutrients in herbal teas. They also help to curb your appetite between meals.

Alfalfa. Chock-full of nutrition and essential amino acids for strength, it's a cleanser and mild laxative to keep your intestinal tract in fit condition. Blend alfalfa with peppermint for a minty flavor and soothing effect.

Bladderwrack. A thyroid tonic and gentle metabolic stimulant to help your body utilize nutrients and burn calories better.

Dandelion. A cleanser and natural diuretic with potassium and vitamins. It prevents constipation and bloating. Unlike standard diuretics that lead to potassium losses that leave you feeling weak, dandelion works gently and naturally to balance your body fluids.

Marigold. A calming floral tea that eases digestive tract disorders and de-stresses your stomach lining and bowels.

Oatstraw. A full body tonic from the oat plant that gives us oat bran and oatmeal. It has lots of vitamins and minerals for staying power.

Papaya. The tropical tea from the melon tree is the one to take instead of antacids. It has an alkalizing enzyme to counteract acidity. It also has enzymes to digest proteins and carbohydrates.

Raspberry. Use iced fruit and berry teas instead of

diet sodas and you'll get fit faster, with herbal energy.
They're rich in vitamins and minerals.

Rosemary. The herb of love and remembrance aids
the digestion of fats, enhances your circulation, and is
good for your heart.

Sage. Increases digestive enzymes and stimulates
your liver to give you new vigor. It's the herb of longevity.

Sweet Treats—Vanilla, Anise, Licorice. Tame those
sugar urges with sweet-treat teas. They curb your appetite and satisfy cravings, while they improve your health.
Natural vanilla is a mood elevator and antioxidant that
can be used as a tea or added to any tea for sweetness.
Anise calms restless digestion and soothes your stomach.
Licorice is a digestive regulator and booster for nutrient
assimilation.

Yerba Mate. A vitality tea with lots of B vitamins to
combat stress. It's a metabolic stimulant that helps your
body utilize carbohydrates, fats, and proteins. Need extra
energy to stay slim? Take yerba mate to the gym.

Healing Waters for Your Bath

Herbal waters for luxurious baths are as close as your
tea closet. Herbal teas are pure botanical waters without
dyes, artificial perfumes, or additives. Since your skin is
also a transmitter of substances, the herb's virtues are
absorbed into your body through your skin.

Recipe: two tea bags per bath. Pour the hot tea into
your bath. You can also float the tea bag in your bath—
it's a ready-made aromatherapy sachet.

Dew of the Sea Bath. Rosemary can be found clinging to the cliffs overlooking the Mediterranean Sea. The
morning dew glistening on rosemary's leaves gave the
herb the name *Dew of the Sea.* A rosemary bath soothes

your nervous system and enhances your circulation. It brings blood to the surface of your skin for a rosy glow. Emerge feeling like you went on a Mediterranean holiday.

Menthol Magic Bath. A native of Europe, peppermint is known for its curative nature and refreshing scent. In peppermint waters, every pore is stimulated by menthol. It's like breathing through your skin. Antiseptic peppermint keeps you germ free. It's excellent for dry skin and gives you a clean feeling that is unbeatable.

Secrets of the Sages Bath. Its name means "to heal," and sage waters cool and soothe while they renew your strength. On a hot night, when you feel drained of energy, slip into a sage bath to cool down. In the throes of a feverish cold, sage reduces body heat and helps you breathe easier. Roman soldiers used it for tired, aching feet, after all that marching in the heat.

Ginger Therapy Bath. On a cold, damp night, when nothing is going right, slip into a ginger bath. It warms you all over, cleanses and purifies your skin. It's like a hydrotherapy treatment for people with cold feet and hands, good for high-stress people who chill easily, or cold feelings that often accompany recovery from an illness.

The Caress of Chamomile Flowers. Indulge yourself in the comfort of a chamomile bath just before bed. It eases aches and pains, and relaxes every muscle in your body. It has the unique ability to soften your skin. A sacred herb in history, the Greeks called it "ground apple" for its charming apple scent.

Thyme Tonic Bath for Your Skin. The scent of balsam will lure you to this treatment for troubled skin. Thyme is a powerful antiseptic for skin conditions—it stimulates blood flow to the area and purges infections. It's antibacterial, antibiotic, antifungal, and antimicrobial to cleanse and heal your skin.

A Modern Medicinal Kitchen: Ten terrific teas to treat you, your family, and friends to the virtues of plants from Heaven

If you are thinking about adding an herbal tea closet to your kitchen but don't know where to start, consider these ten terrific teas. They include some traditional medicinal herbs, some modern favorites, and they represent a well-rounded variety of teas from roots, flowers, leaves, fruits, and whole plants. They will treat many disorders, help to tone your system, and strengthen your resistance to disease.

Astragalus—A root tea with amino acids to restore your immunity, and maintain strong defenses. It also can be used to enhance other teas.

Chamomile—A floral tea to help you unwind at night. It eases stomachaches, soothes your nerves, and lulls you into sleep. It also fights E. coli.

Cranberry—A berry tea for vitamin C, B-complex, iron, and calcium—the antistress nutrients. It also cleanses the urinary tract, bladder, and kidneys.

Dandelion—A root or leaf tea for toning your liver and removing toxins. It's a natural diuretic with potassium to maintain electrolyte balance.

Echinacea—A root tea for colds, flu, infections, gland swelling, and inflammation. It also can be used as a topical wash for skin infections.

Eyebright—A tea for the computer age; the whole plant eases eyestrain, lifts your spirit, clears your head, and gives you a very calm focus. A great tea to take at the office for late-night meetings.

Peppermint—Known as a cure-all, it's a tea for instant energy. The whole plant eases pain, headaches, and tension. A great tea to take in a thermos for long-distance drives. It reduces stress without putting you to sleep.

Plantain—A leaf tea that detoxifies your blood and is

a decongestant for mucous membranes. It's an excellent tea to keep on hand for emergencies—in case of poisoning or toxic conditions. To clean wounds—plantain tea can be used for a wash or a compress.

Tonic Tea—To strengthen your whole body for vital energy.

Eastern Tonics—ginseng root, dong quai root
Western Tonics—sage leaves, whole plant of rosemary
South American Tonics—suma root, yerba mate leaves

The Tenth Tea? Your special needs tea is the one to add that perfect finishing touch to your modern medicinal kitchen.

❧ 5 ❧

Herbal Guide to Health

In this A-Z guide you can look up your current health issues, and find the names of herbs that are most effective for at-home treatment.

To find out more about each herb in the category for your health issues, you'll find profiles of the herbs in Chapter 6, **A Modern Herbal Tea Garden**. There, you will be informed about each herb, its history of use, and given guidance so that you can become a smart consumer of herbs.

What You Can Expect From Your Herbal Guide to Health

The herbs in the A-Z guide were screened to these requirements:

1. The best herbs to take for a particular disorder.
2. The best herbs to take generally.
3. The most recommended herbs in herbal medicine tradition, by current herbals and herbal doctors, re-

search, scientific studies, and other resources that provide guidance for taking herbs.

Take a little time and look up each herb that is listed in the category for your health issues. That way, you can compare the benefits and cautions for each herb in the category, and discover for yourself characteristics that might be particularly suitable or unsuitable for you. In the end, the time you invest in learning about an herb before you use it is an investment in your health. It not only saves you mistakes, it gets you the best remedy.

ABSCESSES
    Burdock
    Calendula
    Echinacea
ACHES, BODY
    Chamomile
    Cramp Bark
    Hyssop
    Marshmallow
ACIDITY, ACID REFLUX
    Catnip
    Chamomile
    Lemon
    Meadowsweet
    Papaya
    Pau d'Arco
    Plantain
    Slippery Elm
    Spearmint
    Yerba Mate
ACNE, BLEMISHES
    (see also Skin Health)
    Calendula
    Echinacea

    Goldenseal
    Lavender
    Oatstraw
    Red Clover
    Thyme
    Yellow Dock
ADRENAL GLANDS, HEALTH
    Astragalus
    Ginseng
    Licorice
    Rose Hips
    Wild Yam
    Yerba Mate
AGITATION
    Passion Flower
    Scullcap
AIDS
    (see Immune Deficiency Disease)
AIR PURIFIER
    Eucalyptus
    Lavender
    Thyme

ALCOHOL WITHDRAWAL
  Milk Thistle
  Passion Flower
  Scullcap

ALLERGIES
  Elder
  Eyebright
  Feverfew
  Ginkgo
  Hyssop
  Lemon Balm
  Milk Thistle
  Parsley
  Thyme

ALZHEIMER'S DISEASE
  Ginkgo

ANEMIA
  Dandelion
  Hawthorn
  Oatstraw
  Pau d'Arco

ANKLES, SWOLLEN
  Butcher's Broom
  Dandelion
  Fennel

ANOREXIA
  Blessed Thistle

ANXIETY
  Hops
  Kava Kava
  Lemon Balm
  Linden Blossoms
  Rosemary
  St. John's Wort
  Vervain

APHRODISIAC
  Damiana
  Fenugreek
  Ginseng
  Rose Hips
  Suma

APPETITE STIMULANT
  Blessed Thistle
  Ginger
  Saw Palmetto

ARTERIES
  Hawthorn
  Lemon
  White Oak

ARTHRITIS
  Alfalfa-Peppermint
  Chamomile
  Cinnamon
  Dong Quai
  Feverfew
  Ginger
  Juniper Berries
  Nettle
  White Willow
  Wild Yam
  Wood Betony

ASTHMA
  Feverfew
  Ginkgo
  Green
  Hyssop
  Lemon Balm
  Lungwort
  Nettle
  Parsley
  Plantain

Thyme
Yerba Santa

Athlete's Foot
Goldenseal
Juniper Berries
Thyme

Balding
Rosemary
White Oak Bark
Yarrow

Bed Wetting
(see Incontinence)

Birth Control Pills
Withdrawal
Chaste Berry
Dong Quai

Bladder Irritation
Chamomile
Dandelion
Echinacea
Marshmallow
Uva Ursi
Yarrow

Blemishes
(see Acne)

Blood Building
Astragalus
Dong Quai
Hawthorn
Nettle
Pau d'Arco
Rose Hips

Blood Cleanser
Burdock
Plantain

Sarsaparilla
Yarrow

Blood Clots
Butcher's Broom
Dong Quai
Ginger

Blood Pressure
Ginger
Ginseng
Green
Hawthorn
Yarrow

Blood Sugar
Burdock
Ginseng
Green
Marshmallow
Sage

Blood Vessels
Feverfew
Sage

Body Odor
Peppermint
Spearmint

Boils
Burdock
Dandelion
Echinacea
Milk Thistle
Slippery Elm

Bone Health
Black Cohosh
Dong Quai
Green
Horsetail
Sarsaparilla

BOWEL INFECTIONS
   Calendula
   Echinacea
   Slippery Elm
BOWEL REGULATOR
   Flax
   Slippery Elm
BRAIN HEALTH
   Ginkgo
   Ginseng
   Gotu Kola
   Parsley
   Rosemary
   Wood Betony
BREATH, BAD
   Anise
   Peppermint
   Spearmint
BREATHING DIFFICULTIES
   Eyebright
   Horehound
   Hyssop
   Lungwort
   Peppermint
   Plantain
BRONCHIAL DILATOR
   Green
   Thyme
BRONCHIAL SPASMS
   Rosemary
BRONCHITIS, BRONCHIAL HEALTH
   Echinacea
   Hyssop
   Horehound
   Lungwort

   Marshmallow
   Peppermint
   Rosemary
BRUISES
   Lavender
   Rose Hips
BURNS
   Aloe
   Chamomile
   Wild Strawberry
BURSITIS
   Horsetail
   Parsley
   White Willow
CANCER
   (see Immunity, General)
CANDIDA
   (see Yeast Infections)
CANKER SORES
   Goldenseal
   Raspberry
CELLULITE
   Dandelion
   Dong Quai
   Ginger (warming)
   Ginkgo
   Gotu Kola
   Hawthorn
   Nettle
   Rose Hips
   Rosemary
   Wood Betony
CHEMOTHERAPY RECUPERATION
   Astragalus
   Milk Thistle

(see Recuperation From
Illness)

"Chi" Tonic
Bitter Orange
Dong Quai
Oatstraw
Schizandra

Chickenpox
Burdock
Calendula
Cleavers

Chills
Cinnamon
Ginger

Cholesterol Regulation
Ginger
Ginseng
Green

Cigarette Withdrawal
(see Nicotine
Withdrawal)

Circulation
Blessed Thistle
Butcher's Broom
Sage
Thyme
Yerba Santa

Cold Hands and Feet
Cinnamon
Ginger

Colds
Echinacea (onset)
Elder
Ginger/Peppermint
Goldenseal (chronic)

Lemon
Plantain (congestion)

Colic
Lavender
Lemon Balm
Peppermint

Colitis, Spastic Colon
Goldenseal
Hops
Marshmallow
Pau d'Arco
Plantain
Slippery Elm

Concentration
Ginkgo
Gotu Kola
Rosemary
Sage

Congestion, Chest
Elder
Hyssop
Peppermint
Plantain
Thyme

Congestion, Nasal
Hyssop
Peppermint
Thyme

Conjunctivitis
Eyebright
Goldenseal
Horsetail
Red Clover

Constipation
Dandelion
Fennel

Papaya
Slippery Elm

CONSTIPATION, STUBBORN
Aloe/Peppermint
Cascara Sagrada
Senna

CONVALESCENCE
(see **Recuperation**)

COUGHS
Anise
Elder
Peppermint
Red Clover
Slippery Elm
Wild Cherry

CRAMPS
Black Cohosh
Chamomile
Cramp Bark

CYSTS
Calendula
Echinacea
Marshmallow
Slippery Elm
Uva Ursi

CYSTITIS
Astragalus
Chamomile
Dandelion
Marshmallow
Pau d'Arco
Slippery Elm
Uva Ursi

DANDRUFF
Catnip Rinse
Sage Rinse

DEPRESSION
Ginseng
Lavender
Lemon Balm
Milk Thistle
Oatstraw
Rose Hips
St. John's Wort
Vervain

DETOXIFIER
Dandelion
Plantain
Yarrow

DIABETES, NON-INSULIN-DEPENDENT
Bilberry
Fenugreek
Marshmallow

DIARRHEA
Bilberry
Raspberry

DIGESTIVE DISORDERS/DISTRESS
Alfalfa/Peppermint
Anise
Bitter Orange
Catnip
Dong Quai
Fennel
Fenugreek
Feverfew
Hops
Meadowsweet
Papaya
Slippery Elm
Yarrow

DIURETIC
Dandelion

DIVERTICULITIS
Fenugreek
Pau d'Arco
Slippery Elm

DIZZINESS
Ginger
Ginkgo
Lavender
Peppermint

DRUG WITHDRAWAL
Catnip
Milk Thistle
Scullcap

DYSENTERY
Bilberry
White Oak
White Willow

EAR CONGESTION
Fenugreek
Ginkgo

ECZEMA
Cleavers
Goldenseal
Red Clover
Wild Strawberry
Yellow Dock

E. COLI FIGHTER
Calendula
Chamomile
Cinnamon
Cranberry
Lemon Grass
Peppermint
Plantain

St. John's Wort
Uva Ursi
Wild Strawberry
Yarrow

EDEMA
Butcher's Broom
Dandelion

ENZYME BOOST
Fennel
Fenugreek
Feverfew
Ginger
Papaya

ESTROGENS
Black Cohosh
Blue Cohosh
Calendula (mild)
Fennel (mild)
Fenugreek
Hops
Licorice
Red Clover

EXPECTORANT
Elder
Horehound
Hyssop
Mullein
Plantain
Rose Hips
Yerba Santa

EYES
Eyebright
Goldenseal
Horsetail
Meadowsweet

EYES, VISION
  Bilberry
  Fennel
  Valerian
FAINTING
  Lavender
FATIGUE
  Astragalus
  Ginseng
  Milk Thistle
  Oatstraw
  Pau d'Arco
  Rose Hips
  Saw Palmetto
  Slippery Elm
  Suma
  Yerba Mate
FEVER
  Burdock
  Echinacea
  Lavender
  Lemon
  Yarrow
FIBROIDS
  Horehound
  Hyssop
  Yellow Dock
FLATULENCE
  (see Gas)
FLU
  Calendula
  Echinacea
  Elder
  Lemon Balm
  Thyme

FLUID BALANCE
  Astragalus
FLUID RETENTION
  Dandelion
FRACTURES
  Comfrey
FRECKLES
  Elder
FREE RADICAL PROTECTION
  Dandelion
  Ginseng
  Green
  Milk Thistle
  Parsley
  Rose Hips
  Rosemary
  Sage
FUNGAL INFECTIONS
  Goldenseal
  Pau d'Arco
  Thyme
GALLBLADDER
  Dandelion
  Parsley
  Peppermint
GALLSTONES
  Dandelion
GAS (FLATULENCE)
  Anise
  Catnip
  Cinnamon
  Fennel
  Papaya
  Peppermint
GASTRIC DISTRESS
  Licorice

Meadowsweet
Papaya
Slippery Elm

GLANDS
(see Lymph System)

GONORRHEA
Cleavers
Pau d'Arco

GOUT
Hawthorn
Juniper Berries
Sassafras
Wild Strawberry

GRAVEL
Fennel
Horsetail

GROWTHS
Milk Thistle
Slippery Elm

GUM DISORDERS
Fennel
Green

GUMS, BLEEDING
Horsetail
Raspberry

GUMS, INFECTIONS
Thyme

GUMS, SPONGY
Vervain
White Oak Bark

HAIR HEALTH
Horsetail

HAIR LOSS
Rosemary
White Oak Bark
Yarrow

HANGOVER
Plantain
Sassafras

HAY FEVER
Elder
Eyebright
Parsley
Thyme

HEADACHES
Feverfew
Ginkgo
Lavender
Milk Thistle
Parsley
Peppermint
Rosemary
Wood Betony

HEART, ARRHYTHMIA
Hawthorn
Rosemary

HEART HEALTH
Astragalus
Calendula
Dong Quai
Ginger
Ginkgo
Hawthorn
Motherwort

HEART PALPITATIONS
Ginseng
Hawthorn
Linden Blossoms
Motherwort
Peppermint

HEART RATE
Hawthorn

HEARTBURN
Catnip
Cinnamon
Peppermint
Sage
Slippery Elm

HEMORRHAGING
Horsetail

HEMORRHOIDS
Butcher's Broom
Goldenseal
Horsetail
Plantain
Yarrow

HEPATITIS
Dandelion
Milk Thistle
Wild Strawberry

HERPES SIMPLEX
Calendula
Hyssop
Juniper Berries
White Oak

HICCOUGHS
Spearmint

HORMONE BALANCE
Astragalus/Dong Quai
Chaste Berry
Gotu Kola
Saw Palmetto

HYPERTENSION
Hawthorn
Siberian Ginseng
Suma

HYPOGLYCEMIA
Dandelion
Yarrow

HYSTERIA
Hops
St. John's Wort
Valerian

**IMMUNE DEFICIENCY
DISEASE, ACQUIRED**
Astragalus
Echinacea
Pau d'Arco
St. John's Wort

IMMUNITY
Astragalus
Echinacea
Ginkgo
Ginseng
Green
Marshmallow
Oatstraw
Pau d'Arco
Rose Hips
Suma

IMPETIGO
Goldenseal

IMPOTENCE
Ginseng
Sarsaparilla
Saw Palmetto

INCONTINENCE
Damiana
Horsetail
St. John's Wort

INDIGESTION
Anise

Bitter Orange
Catnip
Dandelion
Fenugreek
Lemon Verbena
Licorice
Papaya
Sage

INFLAMMATION
Calendula
Dong Quai
Licorice
Marshmallow
Meadowsweet
White Willow

INSOMNIA
Catnip
Chamomile
Hops
Lemon Balm
Licorice
Passion Flower
Valerian

INSULIN PRODUCTION
Dandelion

INTERFERON PRODUCTION
Astragalus
Echinacea

INTESTINAL HEALTH
Bilberry
Burdock
Flax
Marshmallow
Pau d'Arco
Slippery Elm

IRRITABLE BOWEL SYNDROME
Chamomile
Hops
Wild Yam

JAUNDICE
Calendula

JITTERS
Scullcap

JOINTS, CALCIFICATION
Burdock
Dong Quai

JOINTS, STIFFNESS, PAIN
Dong Quai
Hyssop
Yarrow

KIDNEY HEALTH
Cranberry
Damiana
Hawthorn
Horsetail
Marshmallow
Plantain
Raspberry

KIDNEY STONES
Bitter Orange
Cleavers
Horsetail

LARYNGITIS
Fennel
Lavender
Marshmallow
Peppermint

LARYNX INFLAMMATION
Marshmallow
Yerba Santa

LAXATIVE
  Alfalfa
  Cascara Sagrada
  Flax
  Senna
  Yellow Dock
LEARNING IMPAIRED
  Gotu Kola
LIBIDO, BOTH SEXES
  Damiana
  Ginseng
  Sarsaparilla
  Saw Palmetto
  Schizandra
  Yerba Mate
LICE
  Lavender
LIVER HEALTH
  Dandelion
  Dong Quai
  Milk Thistle
  Parsley
LONGEVITY
  Ginkgo
  Ginseng
  Wild Yam
LOWER BOWEL
  INFLAMMATORY
  Calendula
  Slippery Elm
LUMBAGO
  White Willow
LUNGS, HEALTH
  Ginkgo
  Horehound
  Hyssop

Lungwort
Mullein
Plantain
Yerba Mate
LUPUS
  Goldenseal
  Pau d'Arco
LYMPH GLANDS, HEALTH
  Calendula
  Cleavers
  Echinacea
  Papaya
  Pau d'Arco
  Yellow Dock
LYMPH GLANDS, SWOLLEN
  Calendula
MAGNETISM
  Horsetail
MEASLES
  Burdock
  Calendula
  Cleavers
  Goldenseal
MEMORY
  Gingko
  Gotu Kola
  Hawthorn
  Rosemary
  Sage
MENINGITIS
  Goldenseal
MENOPAUSE
  Blessed Thistle
  Black Cohosh
  Chaste Berry
  Dong Quai

Motherwort
Sage
Sarsaparilla
Suma
Wild Yam

MENSTRUATION, DISORDERS
Motherwort

MENSTRUATION, HEAVY BLEEDING:
Goldenseal
Yarrow

MENSTRUATION, REGULATION
Chaste Berry
Dong Quai

MENSTRUATION, SUPPRESSED
Blessed Thistle
Feverfew

METABOLISM
Bladderwrack
Ginger
Sarsaparilla

MIGRAINES
Feverfew
Lavender

MOOD SWINGS
Dandelion
Lavender
Nettle

MOTION SICKNESS
Ginger
Peppermint
Spearmint

MOUTH SORES
Bilberry
Goldenseal
Thyme

MUCOUS CONDITIONS
Goldenseal
Plantain
Slippery Elm

MUSCLE ACHES, TENSION
Chamomile
Cramp Bark
Hyssop
Marshmallow
St. John's Wort
Wild Yam

MUSCLE TONE
Damiana
Dong Quai
Fenugreek
Marshmallow
Raspberry
Suma

MULTIPLE SCLEROSIS
Oatstraw
Pau d'Arco

NAIL FUNGUS
Goldenseal
Thyme

NAILS, HEALTH
Horsetail

NASAL INFECTION
Bayberry
Goldenseal
Thyme

NAUSEA
Ginger
Peppermint
Spearmint

NERVES, NERVOUS TENSION
Damiana
Hops
Lavender
Motherwort
Passion Flower
Peppermint
Rose Hips
Rosemary
Saw Palmetto
Scullcap
St. John's Wort

NERVE PAINS
St. John's Wort

NERVOUS DISORDERS, ALL
Motherwort
Scullcap
St. John's Wort

NEURALGIA, NEURITIS
Black Cohosh
Motherwort
St. John's Wort
White Willow
Wood Betony

NICOTINE WITHDRAWAL
Catnip
Milk Thistle
Scullcap

NIGHT BLINDNESS
Bilberry

NIGHT SWEATS
Sage

NOSEBLEED
Horsetail
Yarrow

OBESITY, OVERWEIGHT
Bladderwrack
Fennel
Papaya
Rosemary
Saw Palmetto

OVARIES, HEALTH
Mullein

PAIN, GENERAL
Black Cohosh
Chamomile
Cramp Bark
Hops
Lavender
Lemon Balm
Passion Flower
Valerian

PANCREAS, HEALTH
Uva Ursi

PANIC
Scullcap

PARASITES
Aloe
Black Walnut
Cleavers
Pau d'Arco
Thyme

PELVIC INFECTIONS
Calendula
Pau d'Arco

PEPTIC ULCERS
Chamomile

PHLEGM
Elder
Feverfew
Goldenseal

Horehound
Hyssop
Plantain
Rose Hips

PINK EYE
Chamomile
Goldenseal

PITUITARY HEALTH
Burdock
Ginseng
Gotu Kola

PMS
Catnip
Chaste Berry
Dong Quai
Hops
Motherwort
Raspberry

PMS HEADACHES
Feverfew

PNEUMONIA
Ginger
Lavender
Papaya
Sage
St. John's Wort
Strawberry
Thyme
Uva Ursi

POISONS, ANTIDOTE
Dandelion
Milk Thistle
Plantain

POISON IVY
Plantain

PROGESTERONE
Sarsaparilla
Wild Yam

PROSTATE PROBLEMS
Buchu
Dandelion
Pau d'Arco
Plantain
Saw Palmetto

PROTEIN DEFICIENCY
Burdock
Fenugreek
Marshmallow
Slippery Elm
Suma

PSORIASIS
Cleavers
Pau d'Arco
Red Clover
Sarsaparilla
Yellow Dock

RADIATION BURNS
Aloe

RADIATION RECUPERATION
Astragalus
Echinacea
(see Recuperation From
Illness)

RASHES
Goldenseal
Thyme

RECUPERATION FROM
ILLNESS
Astragalus
Echinacea
Ginkgo

Green
Marshmallow
Meadowsweet
Milk Thistle
Oatstraw
Rose Hips
Sage
Slippery Elm
Wild Strawberry

RESPIRATORY DISORDERS
Eyebright
Goldenseal
Hyssop
Thyme

RHEUMATISM
Black Cohosh
Bladderwrack
Blue Cohosh
Burdock
Cinnamon
Dandelion
Dong Quai
Hyssop
Lemon
Meadowsweet
White Willow
Wild Strawberry

RINGWORM
Goldenseal
Pau d'Arco
Plantain
Thyme

SALICYLATES
Black Cohosh
Chamomile

Meadowsweet
White Willow Bark

SALMONELLA
Bilberry
Goldenseal
Thyme

SCABIES
Pau d'Arco
Plantain

SCALP, DRY, ITCHY
Juniper Berries

SCALP, STIMULANT
Rosemary

SCIATICA
Feverfew
St. John's Wort
Wood Betony

SEASICKNESS
Ginger
Peppermint
Spearmint

SEBORRHEA
Cleavers
Goldenseal

SEDATIVE
Catnip
Hops
Lemon
Motherwort
Mullein
Passion Flower
Vervain

SHINGLES
Plantain
Sarsaparilla

Sinus Congestion
Bayberry
Fenugreek
Feverfew
Goldenseal
Plantain
Thyme

Skin Health
Calendula
Cleavers
Echinacea
Hops
Lavender
Oatstraw
Red Clover
Rose Hips
Thyme
White Willow

Skin Repair, Tissues
Horsetail
Lavender
Oatstraw

Skin Softener
Chamomile
Echinacea
Marshmallow

Sleep
(see **Insomnia**)

Spinal Nerves, Health
Goldenseal
Motherwort
Yerba Mate

Spirit Lifters
Eyebright
Lemon Balm
Milk Thistle

Peppermint
Rose Hips
Yarrow

Spleen, Health
Fennel
Ginger
Milk Thistle
Pau d'Arco
Uva Ursi
White Oak Bark

Sprains
Comfrey
Vervain

Stamina
Alfalfa/Peppermint
Burdock
Ginseng
Schizandra
Yerba Mate

Steroid Withdrawal
Astragalus
Borage
Licorice
Wild Yam

Stomach Discomfort
Anise
Dong Quai
Fennel
Fenugreek
Papaya
Peppermint

Stomach Inflammation
Calendula
Slippery Elm

Strength
Alfalfa/Peppermint

Borage
Fennel
Oatstraw
Pau d'Arco

STREPTOCOCCUS
Blessed Thistle
Calendula
Ginger
Ginkgo
Horsetail
Lavender
Licorice Root

STRESS
Catnip
Ginseng
Kava Kava
Licorice
Peppermint
Vervain
Yerba Mate

STROKE
Ginkgo

SUNBURN
Aloe
Chamomile
Wild Strawberry

SWEATING
Sage

TEETH, HEALTHY
Green

TENNIS ELBOW
St. John's Wort

TENSION
(see Nervous Tension)

TESTES HEALTH
Mullein
Saw Palmetto

TESTOSTERONE
Damiana
Sarsaparilla

THROAT INFLAMMATION
Bilberry
Elder
Lavender
Marshmallow
Thyme

THROAT, SORE
Bilberry
Elder
Goldenseal
Lavender
Thyme

THRUSH
Bayberry
Goldenseal

THYROID HEALTH
Bladderwrack
Gotu Kola
Oatstraw

TISSUE REPAIR
Horsetail
Marshmallow

TONSILITIS
Elder
Sage
Thyme

TOOTHACHE
Peppermint

TRANQUILIZER
Chamomile

Kava Kava
St. John's Wort
Valerian
TREMORS
Motherwort
TUMORS
(see Immunity)
TWITCHING
Passion Flower
Scullcap
ULCERS
Goldenseal
Horsetail
Licorice
Papaya
Slippery Elm
URETHRITIS
Uva Ursi
URIC ACID BUILDUP
Burdock
Uva Ursi
Vervain
URINARY STONES
Dandelion
Fennel
URINARY TRACT INFECTIONS
Bilberry
Cleavers
Cranberry
Dandelion
Horsetail
Raspberry
Rose Hips
Saw Palmetto
Thyme
Uva Ursi

URINATION, PAINFUL
Horsetail
Juniper Berries
Marshmallow
Uva Ursi
VAGINAL INFECTIONS
Goldenseal
Juniper Berries
Pau d'Arco
VARICOSE VEINS
Ginkgo
Wood Betony
Yarrow
VENEREAL DISEASE
Sarsaparilla (Indian)
White Oak Bark
VERTIGO
Blessed Thistle
Gingko
Rosemary
Wood Betony
VIGOR
Butcher's Broom
Ginseng
Gotu Kola
Pau d'Arco
Rose Hips
Yerba Mate
VIRUSES
Calendula
Cinnamon
Dong Quai
Echinacea
Goldenseal
Green
Lemon Balm

Pau d'Arco
St. John's Wort

VISION
(see Eyes)

VITALITY
Dong Quai
Ginseng
Milk Thistle
Oatstraw
Rosemary
Suma
Yerba Mate

VOMITING
Chamomile
Lavender
Plantain

WEATHER TOLERANCE
Astragalus
Ginger (warming)

WEIGHT CONTROL
Alfalfa
Dandelion
Ginger
Papaya
Rosemary
Saw Palmetto

WORMS
Aloe

Feverfew
Hops
Horehound
Slippery Elm
Thyme

WOUNDS
Aloe
Goldenseal
Horsetail
Slippery Elm
Yarrow

YEAST INFECTIONS
Blessed Thistle
Chaste Berry
Cinnamon
Cleavers
Dong Quai
Ginger
Goldenseal
Parsley
Pau d'Arco
Rosemary
Sage
Thyme
White Oak Bark

❧ 6 ❧

A Modern Herbal
Tea Garden

When you get to know the true nature of herbs, you'll
find that they are down-to-earth bounty from the garden,
with lore and legends that reveal their healing properties.

A Modern Herbal Tea Garden provides you with several tools you can use to be an informed consumer of
herbs:

Common Name: Each profile contains the common
name of the herb, and where appropriate, other names in
common use that the herb might be called.

Latin Name: The Latin name of the herb signifies
the official medicinal herb. For instance, there are many
varieties of rosemary, but only *rosemarinus officinalis* is
considered the medicinal herb. This insures that you get
the proper medicinal herb in the event that a Latin name
is used in a list of ingredients for an herbal remedy, instead of the common name. It also protects you from
false claims. An herbal remedy may say it uses a particular herb, and uses its Latin name. You can check that
name against the official medicinal variety to be sure
they match.

The Latin name can be very important if you are seeking additional information about herbs in scientific literature, or surfing the net for more research on a particular herb. In technical literature about herbs, the Latin name is often the only name used. If your search fails to reveal information with the common name of the herb, use the Latin name.

Profiles: Each profile gives you a picture of the herb and its first-best uses. This saves you time and confusion, since many herbs can have similar or common uses, but only certain herbs have the well-rounded nature that might be best for specific uses. For instance, many herbs have mild diuretic properties that help to stabilize your body's fluid balance, but dandelion is a diuretic herb that carries its own potassium, and that protects you from potassium losses. In that instance, dandelion leads the parade of herbs for its diuretic virtue. By focusing on the herb's best uses, you can be more confident in choosing an effective remedy.

Cautions: In the event that an herb may be considered effective, but also has properties that can be unsuitable for certain people, or harmful in high doses, that restriction is provided in the cautionary note at the end of each herb's profile. It is as important to know the reasons for not taking an herb as it is for taking one. When in doubt, choose the most wholesome herb with the fewest cautions (or none), to stay on the safe side of optimum health.

Beneficent Parts: Only certain parts of an herb are used for medicinal purposes, and it varies from herb to herb. By knowing which parts of the herb are used, you can be sure you are getting the right parts in your remedy.

Properties and Values: You may be surprised to discover the rich nutrient content of many herbs. You may also discover certain vitamins, minerals, or properties in an herb that you might not want or need. By knowing the herb's properties and values, you can become a modern herbal consumer who can rely on information, instead of word-of-mouth endorsements or claims. That way, you avoid the pitfalls, and can go for the peaks in your herbal remedy.

So kick off your shoes, make yourself comfortable, and try an invigorating cup of peppermint tea while you explore the wonders in a modern herbal tea garden. In England, peppermint is considered a cure-all.

ALFALFA   *Medicago sativa*
The Herbal Thoroughbred

Indigenous to Arabia, *Al Fal Fa* is a member of the legume family, with small, split leaves; purple flowers like clovers; and unusual spiral pods. It has long roots that reach deep into the soil for minerals.

Arabian horses are among the most prized breeds in the world, and it was through them that alfalfa's virtues were first discovered by the Arabians. When they saw that alfalfa made their horses swift and strong, the Arabians began to take alfalfa themselves. The herb became known as *The Father of All Foods*.

Alfalfa-Mint Tea

Alfalfa is a super brew to use for energy and staying power, and peppermint brings flavor and synergy to the tea. Use one tea bag of alfalfa and one tea bag of peppermint, steep them together, and pour the blend in a tall glass with ice.

Nutrient Tonic. Alfalfa contains eight essential amino acids; vitamins A, E, K, B, D; phosphorus; iron; potassium; chlorine; sodium; silicon; magnesium; and beta carotene.

Fitness and Weight Control. Alfalfa is a natural diuretic and laxative to ease water retention, cleanse your system, improve digestion, and keep your intestinal tract in fit condition. Because of these values, alfalfa has been used as an aid for weight loss.

Vitamin K. Alfalfa is a source of vitamin K, which is necessary for blood clotting, carbohydrate storage, liver vitality, and longevity. Normally, vitamin K is manufactured by your body's intestinal flora as a by-product of digestion and stored for use. Your body only needs small amounts of vitamin K, and there is rarely a lack of it, except in certain circumstances. Habitual use of aspirin, alcohol, or drugs can destroy your vitamin K supply. In addition, lingering intestinal disorders like colitis can hamper your intestinal flora's ability to make vitamin K. Antibiotics can destroy vitamin K along with friendly flora. In these cases, alfalfa tea can give you the tune-up you need.

Caution: This herb is not recommended for people with autoimmune disorders.

Beneficent Part: Leaves

Properties: Vitamins, Protein, Minerals

Values: Nutrient, Laxative, Tonic, Stomactic, Diuretic

☙

ALOE VERA *Aloe barbadenis*
Juice from the Lilies

Aloes are succulent members of the lily family, often called *desert lilies*, with fibrous roots, and pointed, fleshy leaves that produce a gel and juice. They are natives of tropical Africa, where they still grow in the wilds, but aloes also flourish in the West Indies and Mediterranean countries on cultivated aloe plantations designed exclusively for commerce.

There are more than 200 species of perennial aloe, but only aloe vera is considered the true aloe. True aloe produces a yellowish juice that will seep out when a leaf is cut. There is an American version of aloes called *agaves*, which are not true aloes, and are not used medicinally, so check that aloe, if you are buying a houseplant to keep on hand for cuts or burns, as many people do. True aloes need two to three years to produce their juice, so look for a mature plant with spiny teeth running along the edges of the leaves.

The colors of aloe juices differ, according to the locations where the plants are grown and the methods used to extract the juice. Both the gel and juice come from the aloe's leaves. As a rule, the gel is not used internally, but the juice has a long history for internal use.

Constipation (Stubborn) and Digestive Distress. Aloe tea is a well-respected digestive aid, particularly for severe or stubborn cases of constipation. It relaxes the bowels, acts as a stomach tonic, and stimulates the large intestine. It promotes bile flow to help regulate digestion. In India, a tonic wine is made from fermented aloe gel, blended with honey and spices, and used for anemia, poor digestion, and liver disorders. You can make aloe tea with honey and mint, spiced with cinnamon, to have your own tonic.

Moisturizer. Aloe gel is an emollient that helps skin retain its moisture. It has been called *Nature's Best Moisturizer*. In Ancient Egypt, aloe was regarded as a religious plant, and it is said Cleopatra used its gel to protect her skin from the damaging effects of the hot Egyptian sun.

Parasite Purge. Aloe vera is one of the most effective treatments to expel worms or other parasites from the intestinal tract. It's also antifungal.

Radiation Burns and Skin Surgery. Aloe is a healing *stimulant* that is used topically in the United States to speed healing after radiation burns and skin surgery. You can wash burns with cooled aloe tea, or take an aloe bath.

Aloe Sunburn Bath

If you ever get one of those flaming red sunburns, this recipe will save your skin and let you sleep at night. Make 2–4 bags of aloe tea and pour the tea into a cool bath. Soak in the aloe to take out the sting, activate healing, and prevent moisture loss from your skin.

Uses Through the Ages. As far back as the fourth century, aloe was used by Greek physicians to cure everything from constipation to liver problems.

Caution: In high doses, aloe can cause intestinal cramps. For this reason, aloe is often combined with an herb like peppermint, which eases cramping. Prudent use would be to take aloe only for stubborn digestive disorders or an aggressive attack on intestinal bacteria, for a short term only. Aloe is not recommended for internal use by children, pregnant women, or the elderly.

Beneficent Part: Leaves

Properties: Glycosides, Resins, Polysaccharides, Sterols, Gelonins, Chromones

Values: Purgative, Tonic, Wound Healer, Soother-Tissues, Antifungal, Expels Worms and Parasites, Promotes Bile Flow

ANGELICA   *Angelica Archangelica*

This is the European variety of the Chinese angelica—dong quai. Some say angelica was named for the
Archangel Michael, who ministered to Adam after the
fall, but a French legend from the tenth century attrib-
utes angelica's name to the Archangel Raphael, who told
the secrets of angelica to a monk for use in a plague
epidemic. It is one of the time-honored herbs credited
with angelic virtues. (See **DONG QUAI**)

ANISE   *Anisum pimpinella*
Nature's Sweetness

A native of Egypt, Greece, and Turkey, anise is an
annual with bright green feathery leaves and delicate
flowers in yellow or white.

In olden days, when many diseases were called
"evils" and associated with the work of demons or dev-
ils, anise was credited with averting the evil eye. In Japan, anise trees are often planted in temple gardens.

In ancient Greece, anise was used as a spice on
cakes—the dessert that followed a feast. In France,
Spain, Italy, and South America, it flavors after-dinner
cordials. These cultural traditions also have health benefits. After a night of heavy eating, anise eases indigestion
and settles grouchy stomachs.

A Sweet Treat. Anise is sweet, spicy, and aromatic—
an ideal tea to drink when you crave something sweet.
It's also an excellent sweetener to use with a plainer tea,
since it provides health benefits to add to the brew.

Coughs (Hard and Dry). Anise tea has a soothing
mucilage that can ease those dry coughs that never seem

to go away. It's sweet relief for bronchial and asthmatic coughs.

Sluggish Digestion. At bedtime, anise can calm a restless stomach, soothe digestive distress, ease flatulence, and sweeten the breath.

Beneficent Part: Seeds

Properties: Anethol, Choline, Sugar, Mucilage

Values: Stimulant, Carminative, Diuretic, Antiseptic, Antispasmodic

❧

ASTRAGALUS
Astragalus membranaceous
Also called HUANG QI
The Protector

A native of China and Mongolia, astragalus is a perennial member of the pea family. It has a graceful form, spear-shaped leaves with one middle seam, and rows of pea-shaped flowers that dangle from the stem like bells. It has deep, fibrous, medicinal roots for superior immunity. The sweet-natured golden tea of astragalus will help to restore your natural defenses.

Fluid Balance. Astragalus balances body fluids, which helps to stabilize every body process from healthy cell production to toxin elimination.

Heart Tonic. Astragalus strengthens the cardiovascular system, lowers blood pressure, and stimulates circulation to make your heart's job easier.

Immune Energy. Astragalus invigorates your immune responses. It's an herb that can help you recover from exhaustion, illness, surgery, radiation, and chemotherapy. It has been shown to revitalize white blood cells, and stimulate the production of natural antibodies and natural interferon which your body uses to fight diseases. It helps to restore adrenal function, and provide antiviral resistance. If you get fatigued easily, catch every cold or flu that comes around, and struggle with infections that recur, astragalus is the tea to use to fortify your immunity. A stronger immunity is your best weapon against premature aging and disease.

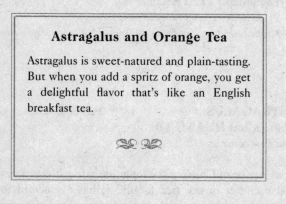

Astragalus and Orange Tea

Astragalus is sweet-natured and plain-tasting. But when you add a spritz of orange, you get a delightful flavor that's like an English breakfast tea.

Protective Energy. In Chinese medicine, astragalus is used to strengthen a unique form of energy that is called "protective energy," which helps us adapt to external factors such as weather changes, and defends us against germs or microorganisms in the environment. They locate this energy beneath the surface of the skin and along the outside of the body—the first line of defense against harmful influences.

Special Feature: Facilitator

Astragalus works like a catalyst to enhance the healing properties of other herbs. When you combine one tea bag of astragalus with one tea bag of your "special needs" herb tea, you get a tonic for energy and renewal. Many herbalists recommend astragalus and dong quai to balance hormonal chemistry in both women and men.

Beneficent Part: Root

Properties: Good Source of Amino Acids, Polysaccharides, Linoleic

Acid, Linolenic Acid, Betaine, Choline, Glycosides, Isoamnitine, Kumatakenin

Values: Tonic, Energizer, Immuno-stimulant, Antimicrobial, Cardiotonic.

❧

BAYBERRY   *Myrica cerifa*
The Germicidal Herb

Bayberry is rich in vitamins and minerals, and has a germicidal agent that fights bacteria and infections. It makes an excellent gargle for sore throats and mouth infections, including thrush, and an effective steam inhalant for sinus congestion.

Caution: Small amounts are advised if bayberry is used in a blend, since bayberry can have a narcoticlike effect in large doses.

Beneficent Part: Root bark

❧

BEARBERRY (see UVA URSI)

❧

BILBERRY   *Vaccinium myrtillus*
The Shrub With Something Special

A native of Europe and Asia, bilberry is a small shrub with angular branches and colorful leaves that change from light red to yellow to vivid red as they season. It blooms with round, waxy flowers and round, black, flat-topped berries. When the berries are ripe, they have a downy gray covering that makes them appear blue.

Dysentery/Diarrhea. This tea is the four-star remedy

for diarrhea and dysentery because it has something special—a pigment that inhibits bacterial growth, especially microorganisms in the intestinal tract which bring on the dysentery and diarrhea. Don't forget to pack bilberry tea bags when you travel! You can drink it on your vacation for intestinal health insurance.

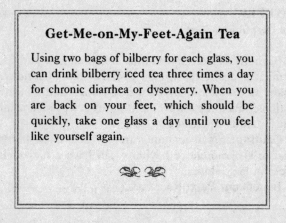

Get-Me-on-My-Feet-Again Tea

Using two bags of bilberry for each glass, you can drink bilberry iced tea three times a day for chronic diarrhea or dysentery. When you are back on your feet, which should be quickly, take one glass a day until you feel like yourself again.

Night Blindness, Computer Eyes, Eyestrain. If you can't adapt to darkness while you're driving, bilberry is the tea you need. Take it routinely to strengthen your vision, defeat eyestrain, and reduce sensitivity to changes in light. It's the herb that Royal Air Force pilots used in World War II to fly night missions.

Non-Insulin-Dependent Diabetes. Research shows that bilberry leaves can increase insulin production and lower blood sugar levels. A tea from the leaves can be beneficial for people with non-insulin-dependent diabetes, when it is used as a routine tea.

Throat Inflammations, Mouth Ulcers. Bilberry tea makes an excellent gargle for inflamed throats and mouth sores, to soothe and heal.

Caution: Avoid bilberry if you take insulin for diabetes.

Beneficent Parts: Fruits and leaves

Properties: Iron, Phosphorus, Potassium, Manganese, Zinc, Fruit Acids, Glycosides, Sugars, Tannins

Values: Antiseptic, Astringent, Diuretic, Lowers Blood Sugar, Prevents Vomiting, Urinary Tract Antiseptic

❧

BLACK (see GREEN)

❧

BLACKBERRY   *Rubus fructicocus*
The Lucky Bramble

This berry bush has its share of folklore that refer to its magic charms. In medieval England, if you wanted to protect yourself from the spells of rheumatism, boils, and blackheads, you'd creep under the bramble bush. To gather the fruits and leaves properly, to insure that they would release their properties, it had to be done at the right time of the moon.

Blackberry, like many berry teas, is astringent and tonic, good for diarrhea and cleansing the system. It's a source of vitamin A, B-complex, and citric and malic acids. A remedy for fevers. The tea can be used to heal bleeding gums. The ancient Greeks used the blossoms to cure gout. Blackberry is often added to blends to bring flavor and harmony.

Beneficent Parts: Root, bark, leaves, berries

❧

BLACK COHOSH
A Sedative Root

Cimicifuga racemosa

Native to shady woodlands of the Eastern United States and Canada, black cohosh has rich green leaves and tall, flowering stems (racemes) covered with white blossoms. Its root is almost black, thick, and knotty.

It has been called *Squaw Root* for its tonic value for women's reproductive tracts, *Rattle Root* and *Black Snake Root* for its use as an antidote to the bites of rattlesnakes.

Neuralgia. A painkiller and sedative that is particularly attuned to pain in muscles and nerves, black cohosh has a long history of use to treat the aches and pains of neuralgia. Low doses are advised, which is a tea in one-half cup servings twice a day.

Rheumatism. Black cohosh has a reputation for successful use as a comforting brew for rheumatism. Its salicylates reduce inflammation, it is antispasmodic to relieve muscle tension, it improves peripheral circulation for better blood flow, and it relieves pain. When rheumatic bouts occur, one-half cup of black cohosh tea in the morning and evening is advised.

Uses Through the Ages. Black cohosh is a uterine tonic and has been used to treat menses pain and delayed periods, since it promotes menstrual flow. In Chinese medicine, black cohosh is used to clear "heat" from the body, reduce toxicity, and relieve asthma, by clearing mucous from bronchial tubes.

Special Feature: Menopause Relief

Black cohosh is one of the herbs that is gaining popularity as a treatment for menopausal symptoms. It is called a phyto-estrogen because of its ability to reduce the levels of LH (pituitary luteinizing hormone), which is believed to be a contributing factor in menopausal symptoms. In European studies, black cohosh combined with St. John's wort was found to relieve menopausal symptoms in 78 percent of the participants. In a study on *surgical menopause*—following a hysterectomy—where the women retained one ovary, black cohosh was found to be comparable to conjugated estrogen. It is estimated that more than five million women in Germany are using black cohosh for menopausal symptoms, along with women from Austria and Scandinavian countries.

Some precautions to consider:

1. Estrogens at Menopause. Estrogenic herbs should not be taken casually for menopausal symptoms, since estrogen supplementation is an individual circumstance for each woman, and it's often not recommended for women with a history of fibrocystic breasts, uterine fibroids, and endometriosis. There are no long-term studies to indicate whether the estrogenlike effects of black cohosh call for the same restraints as synthetic estrogens, but many doctors feel that black cohosh is particularly estrogenic.

2. Hormone Balance. Menopause isn't a measure of a woman's "estrogen" level, it's the balance of progesterone, estrogen, and androgens that needs to be addressed, along with nutrition, exercise, and the whole woman, and it's different for each woman.

3. Low doses are the rule. Black cohosh is a strong herb that should not be taken routinely, and low doses are the rule. In herbal tradition, it was used in small amounts in blends for short-term treatments and pain relief. Menopausal symptoms can last longer than a week or two. For these reasons, seek your doctor's advice if you are considering black cohosh for menopausal symptoms.

Caution: High doses of black cohosh can cause headaches, nausea, and even tremors.

Beneficent Part: Root

Properties: Vitamins A, B1, B2, B3, K, Phosphorus, Calcium, Selenium, Magnesium, Potassium, Iron, Sodium, Silicon, Manganese, Zinc,

Sulfur—Volatile Oil, Triterpene Glycosides, Isoflavones, Isoferalic Acid, Salicylic Acid, Tannins, Resin

Values: Astringent, Alterative, Antispasmodic, Anti-inflammatory, Antirheumatic, Hypotensive, Painkiller, Sedative, Vasodilator, Uterine Tonic, Emmenagogue, Diuretic, Diaphoretic, Mild Expectorant

❧

BLACK WALNUT   *Juglans nigra*
An Infection Fighter

Black walnut has a powerful detergent agent to fight infections, microorganisms, fungus, and parasites. It also has iodine to strengthen the thyroid gland. Since it is a strong detergent, black walnut use is often limited to small amounts in blends to fight infections and strengthen immunity.

Beneficent Part: Bark powder

❧

BLADDERWRACK   *Fucus vesiculosis*
The Thyroid Tonic

This herb is a seaweed that is almost black in color, with ribbons or thalli that are knobby at the joints. It was used in the past as a remedy for swelling of the thyroid from lack of iodine, and in the 18th century, it was a major source of iodine. It stimulates the thyroid and gives your metabolism a gentle kick, for more efficient function. Bladderwrack is rich in minerals and is antirheumatic. The thalli can be used like a dried herb to brew into a healing tea, but you don't need much, it's sea-salty.

Caution: Avoid bladderwrack if you are being treated for a thyroid condition.

Beneficent Part: Thalli

Properties: Mucilage, Minerals, Iodine, Mannitol, Volatile Oil

Values: Metabolic Stimulant, Nutrition, Thyroid Tonic, Antirheumatic, Anti-inflammatory

❧

BLESSED THISTLE
A Special Affinity to Women

Cnicus benedictus
Carduus benedictus

This native of Europe and member of the daisy family has strong stems, spear-shaped leaves with deep center spines and ragged, toothed edges. Called *Holy Thistle* and *St. Benedict's Thistle*, it has been revered for centuries.

Antiaging. Blessed thistle improves circulation, which delivers more oxygen to the brain for memory and alertness, and eases vertigo, dizziness, and headaches.

Cells and Immunity. Blessed Thistle has been credited with antineoplastic virtues and oxygenating value, which can prevent the development of abnormal cells. It is also antibacterial, and its bitters are antimicrobial to give your natural immunity an extra boost.

Women's Life Cycles. Blessed thistle is a valuable aid for menses and menopausal difficulties.

1. Menses. Warm blessed thistle tea helps to bring on a suppressed period, and eases menstrual tension and aches.

2. Menopause. Blessed thistle helps to regulate hormonal balance, and can relieve sudden bouts of bleeding which can occur in menopause.

Special Feature: Appetite Stimulant

Iced blessed thistle tea stimulates the appetite, enhances digestion, and provides essential nutrition to strengthen the body. It's a valuable drink for people who are undernourished or recovering from body-wasting diseases. It has been used to stimulate the appetite for people who have anorexia.

Caution: Moderate use is recommended—one cup of tea per day, and take a break every two weeks.

Beneficent Parts: Whole herb, root, and seeds

Properties: Vitamin A, B-Complex, B3, C, Iron, Magnesium, Phosphorus, Potassium, Sodium, Zinc—Alkaloids, Bitter Principle, Essential Oil, Flavonoids, Mucilage, Tannin

Values: Astringent, Antibacterial, Antiseptic, Diaphoretic, Digestive Aid, Emmenagogue, Expectorant, Stimulant, Tonic

❧

BLUE COHOSH   *Caulophyllum thalictroides*
The Soothing Root

This native of the United States and Canada likes moist places and is at home in swamps or near streams. Its stems and leaves have a purple-blue tint, and it blooms with small purple flowers. It was called *Blueberry Root* for its deep blue berries, *Papoose Root* and *A Woman's Best Friend* for its affinity with the aches and pains of women. It was also called *Blue Ginseng* for its tonic value. Its root is gray-brown and knotty, white inside.

Rheumatism. Blue cohosh is a Native American remedy for rheumatism, with more pain-relieving power than black cohosh. It is often found in small amounts in blends.

Menses. Blue cohosh is a tonic for the reproductive tract, and has been used to treat uterine inflammation and spasms, menses pain, and irregular periods. There is some concern about using blue cohosh for these purposes, since it may inhibit ovulation.

Menopause. Blue cohosh is often cited as one of the menopausal herbs, because of its soothing nature and

steroid-saponins, which are less estrogenic than black cohosh. However, not enough is known about this herb's
full nature to suggest routine or casual intake.

Caution: This herb needs more research and requires
professional guidance for its use. Avoid blue cohosh if
you have heart problems, diabetes, or glaucoma.

Beneficent Part: Root

Properties: Vitamins B1, B2, E, Selenium, Manganese, Iron, Calcium, Magnesium, Phosphorus, Potassium, Silicon, Some Vitamin A and
C, Niacin, Sodium, Chlorine, Zinc

Values: Antispasmodic, Diuretic, Emmenagogue, Demulcent, Sedative, Diaphoretic, Mild Expectorant

❧

BLUE VERVAIN (see **VERVAIN**)
BONESET, a relative of comfrey (see **COMFREY**)

❧

BORAGE   *Borage officinalis*
The Courage and Strength Builder

A native of Europe and England, borage has rough,
dark green leaves, blue star-shaped flowers, and small,
brown, nutlike fruits. The fresh plant has a fragrance like
cucumber, and the leaves have a cucumber taste.

An old adage says that *borage is for courage,* and its
healing properties go straight for the seat of courage—
the adrenal glands.

Courage. Borage stimulates the adrenal cortex—the
"fight or flight" gland that responds to stress. In addition,
borage is a tonic for kidney strength. Strong kidney energy, in Chinese medicine, can help to ease the emotion
fear.

Strength. Borage strengthens the lungs and heart,

and relieves congestion. The tea can help you recover from a period of prolonged fatigue, and fortify your energy reserves during a time of excessive stress or fearfulness. It's also an antidepressant to lift low spirits.

Special Feature: Natural Anti-inflammatory

For inflammatory conditions, borage works better as an iced tea. Borage is best when it is used fresh, not dried.

Caution: Borage contains pyrrolizidine alkaloids which have been linked to liver damage in rats in high doses.

Beneficent Parts: Leaves, flowers, seeds

Properties: Calcium, Potassium, Essential Oil, Mucilage, Pyrrolizidine Alkaloids, Tannins; Seeds Contain Gamma Linoleic Acid

Values: Antidepressant, Anti-inflammatory, Antitoxin, Blood Tonic, Decongestant, Demulcent, Diaphoretic, Diuretic, Galactagogue, Kidney Tonic, Nervine

※

BUCHU   *Barosma betulina*
A South African Charm

Buchu comes from the Cape of Good Hope, and hope is what it brings to men who struggle with prostate enlargement.

Buchu has been called a miracle herb, first brought to Europe in the 17th century, a gift from the Hottentot tribesmen of South Africa. Round buchu *(barosma betulina)* is considered the best. Oval buchu *(barosma crenulata)* is next best. Long buchu *(barosma serratifolia)* has far less volatile oil than the other two.

Prostate Enlargement (Inflammation and Infection). Buchu is a dispersing herb for superior cleansing. It contains a camphorlike oil that kills infections and reduces prostate inflammation. Tribesmen used a special blend of buchu and alcohol for prostate inflammation. Buchu's properties are released best in alcohol, so a tincture can be used to make an iced tea, to be taken twice a day. Follow with plenty of water to wash out toxins.

Caution: Prudent use is recommended to avoid gastrointestinal distress.

Beneficent Part: Leaves

Properties: Camphorlike Oil, Calcium, Iron, Magnesium, Manganese, Phosphorus, Potassium, Selenium, Silicon

Values: Superior Cleanser, Diaphoretic, Aromatic

❧

BUCKTHORN (see CASCARA SAGRADA)

❧

BURDOCK   *Arctium lappa*
The Big Guy of Purifiers

This member of the thistle family is indigenous to roadsides and dry fields in Europe and England. It has large, dark-green, crinkled, ruffle-edged leaves, and blooms in close clusters of small purple-pink flowers.

Blood. Burdock has the best reputation as a blood cleanser. Pioneers ate the roots and leaves raw to keep their blood pure.

Blood Sugar. Burdock tea can help to lower blood sugar levels.

Calcification in Joints. Excess uric acid can lead to calcification in joints, and muscle and joint pain. Burdock is one of the best cleansers for uric acid and wastes—a tea to take for arthritis, rheumatism, lumbago, and sciatica.

Digestion. Burdock has bitters which stimulate and

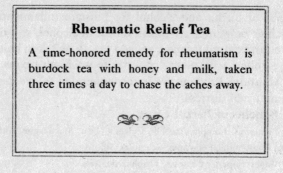

Rheumatic Relief Tea

A time-honored remedy for rheumatism is burdock tea with honey and milk, taken three times a day to chase the aches away.

strengthen your digestive system. It also contains inulin which benefits the liver, spleen, and pancreas.

Glands—Hypothalamus, Pituitary, Lymph, Sebaceous. Burdock cleanses the glands and helps to stabilize their function, including hormone balance by the pituitary. It's an *alterative* herb—one that gently creates positive, healing changes when it is used routinely. It stimulates the sweat glands to remove toxins from the skin, and is mildly diuretic to release toxins through the urine. It also reduces fevers.

Intestinal Health. Burdock is a bear against intestinal disorders. It removes toxins, fights bacteria and fungus, and supports healthy intestinal flora with vital nutrients. It's mildly laxative to keep wastes from stagnating.

Measles, Chickenpox. Burdock is a traditional remedy to speed healing of eruptive infections. It stimulates the glands to remove toxins. For infections, take internally, and use the tea as a topical application on the site of infection. It cools and dries the area, while it fights the infection.

Special Feature: Good source of protein
Beneficent Parts. Roots, seeds, leaves

Properties: High in Protein, Phosphorus, Calcium; also Iron, Magnesium, Potassium, Sodium, Silicon, Selenium, Manganese, Chromium,

Cobalt, Zinc, Inulin, Vitamins A, B-Complex, C, E, Bioflavonoids, Volatile Acids, Tannins, Polyphenolic Acid, Bitters

Values: Alterative, Antibiotic, Antifungal, Antibacterial, Bitter Tonic, Nutrient Tonic, Digestive Stimulant, Diuretic, Diaphoretic, Hypoglycemic, Mild Laxative

❧

BUTCHER'S BROOM
The Clean Sweeper

Ruscus aculeatus

A native of Europe, butcher's broom is all branches and no leaves. It produces small greenish flowers and red berries. In England, its branches were tied in bundles to use for brooms to clean cutting blocks in butcher shops.

Cleanser. Butcher's broom is one of the best internal cleansers to remove toxins and renew energy. Butcher's broom tea can make a clean sweep through your kidneys and liver (it's good for the prostate too).

Energizer. Butcher's broom is an invigorating, antiaging tea that renews energy by renewing circulation, which provides oxygen to the body and brain. It also strengthens muscles and blood vessels, and it "moves" blood to relieve stagnation.

Swollen Legs and Ankles. Butcher's broom boosts circulation—especially in the legs. It is used to prevent fluid retention in the legs and ankles, often called edema.

Uses Through the Ages. Studies in France showed that butcher's broom significantly reduced the incidence of clotting after surgery.

Beneficent Parts: Root and seeds

Properties: Vitamins B1, B3, C, Calcium, Iron, Manganese, Potassium, Selenium, Sodium, Zinc

Values: Circulatory Tonic, Diuretic, Diaphoretic, Oxygenator, Energizer, Anti-inflammatory

CALENDULA (MARIGOLD) *Calendula officinalis*

A Pot of Gold

Calendula, or *Pot Marigold*, was native to the Canary Islands and the Mediterranean shores, but rapidly became a world-favorite herb. It's a hardy annual with sturdy stems and full green leaves that are clearly veined and curve slightly. It blooms all summer with ruffle-edged flowers in golden yellow or orange. They add a special kind of cheer to any garden.

Legend of the Sun Followers

Calendula is one of the earliest medicinal plants, loved by gods and goddesses, mothers, and other healers. Greek myth claims that the flowers weren't always grounded. Once, they were nymphs of the forest.

All of the wood nymphs on Mount Olympus adored the sun god, Apollo. Among the nymphs, four tended Apollo's twin sister Artemis, the goddess of the moon and forest. These four nymphs were so love struck with Apollo, they quarreled constantly, and vied with each other for his attention. One day, Artemis found them arguing about her brother again, and to end their rivalry forever, she turned the nymphs into calendula flowers.

The gold flowers traveled the trade routes and attracted attention wherever they went. They were exchanged for black tea in the Far East. In ancient Rome, where yellow was a symbol of luxury, calendula popped up in the richest gardens. In India, calendula was sacred to the goddess Dwiga, and she wears the flowers on her emblem.

In the 13th century, calendula petals were used to "comfort the heart and spirit." In the 16th century, they were used for soups, broths, jams, jellies, and to color butter and cheese. In France, they were called *souci du jardin*—"sauce of the garden," or "sun-follower," and their petals topped gourmet salads. In 1672 in America, a list of "New England Rarities" said that marigolds were thriving in the new world.

In the early days of Christianity, many medicinal plants were adopted into the new religion and given new names. Calendula was called *Marigolde* or *Mary's Gold*, in honor of the Virgin Mary. That name remains to this day as marigold. The tea is also called marigold.

Heart Health. Marigold flower petals mixed with honey have been used as a treatment for weak hearts through the ages. Add honey to your marigold tea and have this drink at your fingertips for healthy heart maintenance.

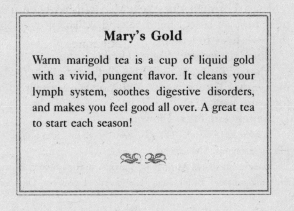

Mary's Gold

Warm marigold tea is a cup of liquid gold with a vivid, pungent flavor. It cleans your lymph system, soothes digestive disorders, and makes you feel good all over. A great tea to start each season!

Inflammations (Digestive Tract). Marigold tea is excellent to ease digestive distress, and soothe inflammatory conditions in stomach lining and bowels.

Lymph Glands. Marigold tea relieves congestion in the lymph system and reduces swollen lymph glands. It improves circulation and detoxifies the body. A great tea to take before flu season.

Menopause. Marigold has estrogenic properties to help to ease the transition from estrogen production in the ovaries to estrogen production by the adrenal glands.

Menstruation. Marigold is beneficial for the female reproductive system to ease menstrual difficulties and regulate menstruation.

Pelvic Infections. Marigold has antibacterial properties that are particularly powerful fungus fighters, for pelvic and bowel infections.

Skin Wash. Two tea bags of marigold in one cup of water makes a potent, pure skin wash. Apply the tea with cotton balls to skin eruptions (even measles and chickenpox) to dry and heal them. It's known as a first-class first-aid remedy for cuts and sores. In English herb shops, it's sold as a wash for skin infections.

Uses Through the Ages. Marigold has been used to treat tumors, cysts, jaundice, and inflamed eyes and to improve liver function.

Special Feature: Fights Herpes Simplex

Marigold is an antiviral tea that can fight herpes simplex virus. Take it warm. You can also use marigold tea for a sitz bath.

Beneficent Part: Flowers

Properties: Essential Oil, Carotenoids, Resin, Flavonoids, Sterol, Bitters, Saponins, Mucilage

Values: Antiseptic, Astringent, Antiviral, Antispasmodic, Estrogenic, Anti-inflammatory, Bitter Tonic, Diaphoretic, Detoxifier, Diuretic

CASCARA SAGRADA
Also called BUCKTHORN
Rhamnus purshiana
A Bitter Tonic Bark

The one- to two-year-old purple-brown bark of this native of California and British Columbia is a bitter tonic and laxative. It was called *The Great Herb* and *Sacred Bark* by the North American Amerind Indians.

Chronic Constipation. Cascara tea brings quick relief from chronic constipation. It gets rid of wastes fast. It stimulates the pituitary gland, is beneficial for the pancreas, liver, spleen, gallbladder, and stomach, and it's a good digestive remedy. It acts on the upper intestinal lining to spur a bowel movement, fights bacteria and gas, tones the intestines and colon, and can help to prevent intestinal diseases that result from stagnant wastes. Depending on the individual, cascara's laxative effect can work in a few hours or overnight. This is a bark with a very bitter taste, and the conservative way to take it is in small amounts in a blend.

Caution: Use sparingly, not more than one or two weeks. Regular use can lead to potassium depletion and diarrhea.

Properties: Laxative Anthraquinones, High in Vitamins A, B-Complex, B1, B2, C, Calcium, Chlorine, Iron, Niacin, Potassium, Phosphorus, Selenium, Silicon, Sodium, Trace Minerals

Values: Laxative, Bitter Tonic, Digestive Stimulant, Calming to Nerves, Nutrients

CATNIP   *Nepeta cataria*
Also called CATMINT
The Antistress Herb

This native of England has hairy stems, gray-green leaves that are downy with hairs, and it blooms with white flowers that are spotted with red.

Acid Reflux. Catnip isn't just for cats. It's a *natural antacid* for stomach distress and acid reflux.

Drug and Nicotine Withdrawal. Catnip tea helps to ease the stress and internal tension that comes from nicotine or drug withdrawal. You can also use it to soothe your system after long periods on prescription drugs.

PMS. Catnip tea is good for cramps and premenstrual tension. An old-time remedy for premenstrual tension was a *catnip bath*. It's an emmenagogue, which means that it will bring on a period that is slow to start.

Stress Relief All Over. Catnip is a marvelous tea for all-over relief. Soothing and sedative for your nerves, it eases internal stress, anxiety, stops internal spasms, soothes digestive distress, fights indigestion, heartburn, and gas.

Soothing Sleep Aid. Catnip tea is a gentle way to achieve more restful sleep.

Special Feature: Dandruff Rinse
Catnip tea is an antidandruff rinse for your scalp.
Beneficent Parts: Flowers and leaves

Properties: Vitamins A, B, C, Calcium, Iron, Magnesium, Manganese, Phosphorus, Potassium, Selenium, Sodium, Silicon

Values: Mild Astringent, Mild Antibiotic, Soothing Sedative, Stomachic, Antispasmodic, Relaxant, Carminative, Emmenagogue

CHAMOMILE

The All-Around Comforter

Roman: *Chamaemelum nobile*
(*Anthemis nobilis*)

German: *Matricaria chamomille*
(*Matricaria recutita*)

There are many varieties of chamomile, but only two are used medicinally—Roman chamomile, a perennial from Europe and the United States, and German chamomile, an annual that is considered a Eurasian species.

Roman chamomile is a perennial that grows close to the ground and forges new trails with branches that can root at their base. Its leaves are gray-green, segmented, and feathery. It blooms in late summer with flowers that resemble miniature white daisies with flat, solid yellow centers. In the United States during the American Revolution, chamomile was called *Whig Plant*, because it grew better when stepped on, and remained upright. In England, chamomile lawns are a landscaping feature—when they are walked on, the herb breaks and fills the air with an applelike fragrance.

German chamomile is an annual herb about two feet in height, with smooth stems, slender branches, and segmented leaves. Bright green leaves alternate on light green stems, and often wrap the stem at their base. Its miniature daisylike flowers have white petals and hollow conical centers. This is thought to be the chamomile from ancient times, and the best chamomile for a nightcap. In Spain, its flowers are used to flavor sherries.

Sacred Apple of the Ground

Chamomile was one of the nine sacred herbs of the Saxons, who called it *maythen*. Its name comes from the

Greek *chamai*—"on the ground" and *melon*—"ground apple," after its fragrance. The French cherish it as one of their six favored *tisanes*, or herb teas, taken not only for social pleasure, but as a natural health custom. It's gentle and caressing.

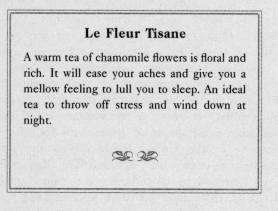

Le Fleur Tisane

A warm tea of chamomile flowers is floral and rich. It will ease your aches and give you a mellow feeling to lull you to sleep. An ideal tea to throw off stress and wind down at night.

Aches, Pains, Cramps. Chamomile tea provides full body relief for muscle aches, strains, arthritic pain, and menstrual cramps.

Bladder Irritation. Chamomile reduces inflammations and helps to fight infections in the bladder. It helps to ease related conditions such as cystitis and fights E. coli in the bladder.

Burns, Scalds. Chamomile is antiseptic and antibacterial for a skin wash or burn bath, and it takes the pain away to help you sleep.

Nausea, Vomiting. Chamomile relieves nausea, relaxes tension, and stops vomiting.

Skin Softer to Touch. Chamomile relaxes tension in your muscles, and softens your skin. Take a chamomile bath tonight with 2–4 bags of tea water and love the skin you're in.

Sleep Ease. It calms, cools, and tranquilizes to help you fall asleep naturally.

Tranquilizer. Relaxes all of the smooth muscles in your body, including the muscles of your digestive tract. Relieves spasms, abdominal pain, bloating, and gas. It regulates peristalsis to prevent diarrhea or constipation. A very beneficial tea for people with disorders that are aggravated by stress, such as irritable bowel, indigestion, gastritis, and peptic ulcers.

Uses Through the Ages. Chamomile has been used to treat eye inflammations, including pink eye. It has also been used as a bronchial relaxant for asthma, hay fever, and sinusitis.

Special Feature: Hair rinse

Chamomile tea as a hair rinse will add highlights to blond hair.

Beneficent Part: Flowers

Properties: Volatile Oil, Flavonoids, Valerianic Acid, Coumarins, Tannins, Glycosides, Salicylates

Values: Antispasmodic, Sedative, Anti-inflammatory, Bitters, Antiseptic, Antibacterial, Prevents Vomiting

❧

CHAPARRAL
Larrea tridentata
A Potent Antioxidant

Chaparral is a vigorous blood cleanser and antiseptic that fights mold, fungus, bacteria, viruses, and infections. It also contains a powerful antioxidant that fights free radical damage. It has expectorant action for respiratory congestion and is a good source of protein, vitamins, and minerals.

Caution: Chaparral has been known to cause severe liver damage. It's a strong herb that shouldn't be used

casually. Seek professional guidance for its use. It can be
found in small amounts in blends.

Beneficent Parts: Leaves and stems

❧

CHASTE BERRY
Vitex agnus castus
Also called VITEX
A Woman's Balance

Chaste Berry is a woman's herb for hormone balance
that stimulates the pituitary gland, and reputedly doesn't
have hormonal properties. It can be used for the roller-
coaster emotions of PMS, irregular periods, menstrual
pain, and to regulate hormones in menopause. It is recommended for use when withdrawing from birth control
pills. It's calming for the emotions.

Beneficent Parts: Berries, leaves, seeds

❧

CHERRY, WILD
Prunus serotina
The Cough Suppressant
Prunus virginiana

Indigenous to North America and the southwestern
United States, wild cherry is an eighty-foot tree with
black bark and oval leaves with small teeth. It blooms
with white flowers and deep purple fruit.

Coughs (Dry) and Congestion. Wild cherry is an antitussive—an herb that relaxes bronchial spasms that initiate coughing. But it doesn't stop there as a treatment
for bronchitis, mucous congestion, lung weakness, dry
coughs, whooping cough, and respiratory disorders. It has
antiseptic properties to fight infections, expectorant action to remove mucous buildup; for stressful respiratory
problems such as colds, flu, and chronic congestion, its

sedative and tranquilizing properties help you get the rest you need to facilitate healing. Wild cherry is often found in small amounts in blends or syrups for bronchial and respiratory disorders.

Caution: Wild cherry is not recommended for regular use or in large doses, since its sedative property, hydrocyanic acid, is toxic in large doses.

Beneficent Part: Root bark and inner tree bark

Properties: Bitter Principle, Sedative, Prunin Resin (antiacidity), Malic Acid

Values: Tonic, Astringent Sedative, Pectoral, Expectorant, Antitussive, Antiseptic

&

CHICORY
Chicorium intybus
A Balancing Herb for Blends

A native of Europe and a roadside member of the dandelion clan, chicory has twiggy stems, angular branches, and bright blue flowers with jagged edges. It's an antiseptic cleanser, laxative, and diuretic to rid your body of uric acid and wastes. It reduces stomach acidity, stimulates the liver, cleanses the spleen, gallbladder, and kidneys. Chicory is a *carminative* herb—one that reduces spasms. It is often used to balance blends of laxatives and cleansers, and to enhance flavor. It's a substitute or ingredient in coffee. It has no caffeine or caffeo-tannic acids, and lots of silica for tissue repair. It has a long history of use as a food. In Belgium, for example, the leaves and roots are eaten as a vegetable. In France, young leaves are used in salads.

Caution: Chicory is not recommended for habitual use, since it can deplete energy and cause weakness in vision.

Beneficent Parts: Leaves and root

❦

CINNAMON
A Spice for Blends

Cinnamon zeylanicum
Cinnamon cassia

Cinnamon is a warm spice with a sweet, calming nature that is used to enhance blends for cold conditions, such as colds, chills, arthritis, and rheumatism. On a cold winter night, when you feel chilled all over, one of the familiar rolled cinnamon sticks can top off your tea while it's steeping. It will warm you as you drink it, and you'll derive some fabulous health benefits. Cinnamon is antiseptic to fight bacteria, viruses, fungal and yeast infections. It's anti–E. coli. It's a digestive aid and anesthetic. All that disease resistance from a simple cinnamon stick used for flavoring!

Beneficent Part: Inner Bark

❦

CLEAVERS
The Lymph Cleanser

Galium aparine
Galium rubiaceae

A native of North America, Europe, and Australia, cleavers can be spotted in gardens and by roadsides as one of the first herbs of early spring. It's a twining weed that weaves through other plants and shrubs with long, square, sticky stems, pinwheels of slim leaves up the stem, and clusters of small white flowers. It produces a small, round, prickly green fruit. Its name comes from its clinging or "cleaving" nature, and it will stick to fabric and people. For this quality, it's been called *Love-man*, *Everlasting Friendship*, *Gripgrass*, *Catchweed*, and *Stickie-willie*.

Lymph Glands (Swollen) and Lymph System Cleanser. This virtue earns cleavers its name *Love-man*.

Lymph cleansing is vital for immunity! It helps to prevent lymphatic buildup and lymph toxins which can contribute to the development of breast cysts, tumors, glandular fevers, prostate infections, and urinary tract infections such as cystitis. The lymph glands also influence conditions of the skin such as eczema, psoriasis, acne, boils, abscesses, and eruptive infections.

The natural way to work on lymph-related difficulties is to cleanse your lymph system at least twice a year—in fall, before cold and flu season, and in spring, to greet the new season with a fresh feeling. Try cleavers tea every day for one week for a lymph cleansing treatment. It drains toxins from the lymph system, reduces swelling of the glands, and can ease congestion in the breasts. It also stimulates the liver, another detoxifying organ, and enhances digestion and absorption of nutrients.

For a super treatment, combine one tea bag of lymph-cleansing cleavers with one tea bag of liver-cleansing milk thistle. That way, lymph debris and liver toxins get out of your system fast. Both cleavers and milk thistle are wholesome herbs and can be taken more often if you need them.

Skin Disorders. Eczema, seborrhea, psoriasis, blemishes, recurring infections, and all skin disorders can be improved with lymph cleansing. Cleavers tea will clean the lymph system to help to resolve these disorders internally. Simultaneously, you can use the tea as a skin wash on the site to treat the problem inside and out. Cleavers is also a cleanser for eruptive infections such as measles and chickenpox.

Uses Through the Ages. In New Zealand, cleavers is used to treat gonorrhea. In Mexico, it is used for intestinal parasites and fevers. It has also been used for kidney stones and urinary troubles. The ancient Greeks used it to treat "weariness," which can result from stagnant liver and lymph.

Beneficent Parts: Leaves, stems, flowers

Properties: Coumarins, Tannins, Glycosides, Citric Acid

Values: Lymphatic Cleanser, Tonic, Nervine, Alterative, Mild Astringent, Diuretic

⁂

COMFREY   *Symphytum official*
An Herb for Repairs

A native of Europe and member of the borage family, comfrey is called a water plant, because it likes riverbanks and moist places. It has a hollow, hairy stem, large hairy leaves that grow smaller as they rise up on the stem, and it blooms from spikes with small white flowers.

Fractures, Sprains, Arthritic Joints. Comfrey has been called *Knitbone* for its ability to repair fractures and restore muscles and tissues. It contains allantoin, which promotes the growth of muscle cells, bone, and cartilage. The tea can be used for a warm compress on the site. Soak a clean cloth in warm comfrey tea and cover the site. This allows the allantoin to be absorbed through the skin to speed healing to the area. If there is also a wound, clean the area thoroughly to prevent debris from being trapped in the site, since comfrey is a rapid healer. A great antiseptic to wash the site is thyme tea.

Uses Through the Ages. These uses might not be tea for two, but they show that some things never change. A 16th century herbal recommends comfrey as a poultice for men with bad backs from "wrestling" or "overmuch use of women." For women, a comfrey bath was a premarital treatment—since it mends rips or tears, comfrey was used to mend the hymen to restore virginity.

Caution: Recent studies show that the pyrrolizidine alkaloids in comfrey have caused liver damage in rats, when administered in high doses. Therefore, the best holistic use for comfrey is topical.

Beneficent Part: Whole plant

Properties: Vitamin B12, Protein, Mucilage, Steroidal Saponins, Allantoin, Tannins, Pyrrolizidine Alkaloids, Inulin

Values: Promotes Cell Growth, Astringent, Demulcent, Wound Healer, Expectorant

☙

CRAMP BARK   *Viburnum opulus*
Also called GUELDER ROSE
The Comforter for Cramps

Cramp bark is a large bush with a gray-brown bark, three-lobed leaves, and snowball clusters of white flowers. It's Mother Nature's remedy for cramps and muscle tension.

PMS. Cramp Bark is a particularly good tea for women who struggle with extreme lower body stress during PMS and menstruation, which can include a cold, heavy feeling in the lower body, abdominal pain, uterine pressure, back pain, bladder distress, leg aches, and fluid retention. Cramp bark is a uterine tonic and sedative with strong antispasmodic properties to relieve backaches, muscle tension, pains in the legs, and bearing-down pressure. It's soothing to the nervous system, and it's a diuretic to relieve bloating and fluid retention. Cramp bark is also calming for the cardiovascular system to ease palpitations. Cramp bark is often found in small amounts in blends. If you take it solo, as purists do, make a weaker tea than usual, and sip it slowly. Sweeten it with honey and lemon for a little extra comfort.

Beneficent Part: Bark

Properties: Bitter Principle, Saponins, Valerianic Acid, Tannins

Values: Antispasmodic, Anti-inflammatory, Astringent, Relaxes Muscle Tension, Sedative

❧

CRANBERRY   *Vacinnium macrocarpan*
The Red Fruit Remedy   *Vacinnium oxycoccus*

Cranberry is native to Europe, Asia, and North America from Alaska to Tennessee. It's a shrub of the evergreen family that thrives in wet and mountainous areas (bogs), with pink-toned stems, oval leaves, and purple or pink flowers in spring. In fall, it produces bright red berries that are popular for Thanksgiving feasts, as sauces, jellies, and decorations.

Urinary Tract Infections. It is estimated that more than fifty million cases of urinary tract infections occur in the United States each year. The majority of cases are women, and standard treatment has been *antibiotics*. But antibiotics aren't the panacea pills anymore. They can create new bacterial strains that resist future antibiotics, and when bacteria is eliminated, antibiotics can attack the lining of the bladder, making it weaker. So they aren't *the best first choice* for resolving urinary tract infections.

Many experts recommend cranberry juice and vitamin C, but it's not the fastest route to healing. Cranberry *juice* contains only ten to thirty percent cranberries, and lots of sugar. Sugary environments support bacteria, so sugar intake needs to be *minimal*. Even if you use unsweetened cranberry juice, the cranberry content is low, and often there are additives. What can you do?

Cranberry tea to the rescue. It's all cranberries, *no sugar*, and it already has vitamin C as one of its virtues. Plain and simple treatment. That's the beauty of teas!

E. Coli Fighter. Urinary tract infections can be spread during intercourse, or they can occur within your own system if bacteria from your intestines get into the urethra canal. Some infections can be viral, but it is estimated that more than 85 percent are due to E. coli bacteria in the urethra canal.

It's important to stop a urinary tract infection in its early stages, because it can spread to your bladder or kidneys in the following way:

Stage 1: E. coli are part of the normal flora in your intestines that help to break down digestive by-products. The trouble begins when E. coli start traveling up the urethral canal, creating irritation. You get a sensation of burning or tension during urination (Urethritis). The urethral canal is connected to the bladder, and if this irritation goes unchecked, the bacteria continue to spread up the urethral canal to the bladder.

Stage 2: E. coli enter the bladder and cling to bladder walls, multiply, and create an infection in the bladder lining. The infection causes inflammation in the lining which can break small capillaries. Blood spots from the capillaries show up in urine (Cystitis). If this infection goes unchecked, E. coli start traveling up the ureter tubes that connect your bladder to your kidneys.

Stage 3: E. coli enter your kidneys and create an infection there. It produces back pain, chills, fever, and nausea.

Women are more vulnerable to bladder infections because their urethral canal is shorter than men's, and straighter. A woman's urethral canal is about three inches long, while a man's is about ten inches long, with bends that make it harder for bacteria to make it all the way to the bladder.

Researchers at Weber State University in Utah found that people with Tamms-Horsfall (T-H) glycoprotein in their urine have fewer bladder infections because this

substance grabs E. coli and keeps it from clinging to
bladder walls. The same researchers found that cranberry
has a substance like T-H glycoprotein that prevents E.
coli from adhering to bladder walls.

Teas for Treatment. Thanks to cranberry tea, you can
keep E. coli bacteria away from bladder walls. Thanks to
antiviral and antibacterial echinacea, you can fight the
infection. And thanks to chamomile, you can sleep com-
fortably, since chamomile fights E. coli *and* inflammation.

3-Tea Treatment for UT Health
Cranberry/Echinacea Blend,
Chamomile at Bedtime

A tea bag of cranberry combined with a tea bag of
echinacea is a potent daytime remedy to boost your immunity and fight E. coli. Take the tea cool or iced, since
UT infections cause inflammation, which is *heat*-produc-
ing. Have your chamomile warm, since it's a bedtime tea.

When your condition improves, forgo the echinacea,
but make cranberry tea part of your weekly health routine for protection. Take the chamomile regularly, if you
prefer.

Cranberry for Lovers

A tall, cool glass of iced cranberry tea might be just
the refreshment you need for those cozy, intimate din-
ners.

Urinary tract infections suggest that your immunity
isn't up to par. To be on the safe side, and fight the
possibility of a recurring bout:

Cranberry + Immunity
Cranberry and Astragalus

One tea bag of astragalus and one tea bag of cranberry makes a tangy, rich tonic for super protection against urinary tract infections. The astragalus boosts your body's immunity and acts as a catalyst to help the cranberry work even better to tone your urinary tract. It's an exhilarating tea!

Beneficent Part: Berries

Properties: Citric and Malic Acid, Quinic, Benzoic Acids, Vitamins A, B-Complex, C, Minerals, Rich in Iron and Calcium

Values: Nutritious Tonic, Toner for Urinary Tract, Bladder and Kidneys, Mild Diuretic

❧

DAMIANA   *Turnera aphrodisiaca*
The Love Potion

Indigenous to Texas, Mexico, South America, and Africa, damiana is a small shrub with pale green, wedge-shaped leaves and a bloom of aromatic yellow flowers. Its name comes from the Greek *aphrodisiakos*, for Aphrodite, the goddess of love. It's a tonic for men and women.

Libido: Damiana acts directly on the reproductive organs. For men, it stimulates testosterone to fight impotence, sterility, and prostate problems. For women, it fights infertility, builds red blood, balances hormones, helps to establish healthy menstrual cycles, and is used in menopause to ease hormonal transitions and hot flashes. But don't expect a rush like wine because it's an aphrodisiac. Herbal aphrodisiacs work on a deeper level to bring harmony to your body. That makes you feel like you're in love with life.

Nerve Tonic: The Love Goddess would never say, "Not tonight, I have a headache." Damiana helps to soothe and strengthen the brain and nervous system which calms the nerves, eases tension headaches, fights exhaustion, and it's even attributed with improving muscular tone and energy. It's also good for the kidneys, to renew energy.

Special Feature: Damiana is known to treat incontinence. A cup of tea in the evening can ease a troubled sleep.

Beneficent Part: Leaves

Properties: Volatile Oil, Resins, Damianin Tannin, Sugar, Albuminoids, Vitamins A, B1, B2, C, Iron, Magnesium, Manganese, Potassium, Phosphorus, Selenium, Silica, Sodium, Zinc

Values: Aphrodisiac, Tonic, Stimulant, Laxative, Mild Purgative, Nutrient Source

❧

DANDELION
Taraxacum officinale
The Little Plant That Roars

This persistent lawn flower is thought of as an annoying weed to many grass lovers, and they yank it perennially, without realizing that they are scrapping an official medicinal plant, packed with nutrients, including vitamins A, B, C, D; iron; and lots of potassium.

It's been called *Priest's Crown*, and its design is virtually a self-watering phenomenon.

It has long, shiny leaves with deep grooves and jagged edges that grow in a circular cluster close to the ground. When rain falls, it travels down the grooves in the leaves to the center, straight to dandelion's tap root from all points round. In spring, a long, hollow, leafless, purple stem rises straight from the root and produces a single bright, golden flower.

Its name is attributed to a surgeon in the 15th century who thought the leaves resembled a lion's teeth, and called it *dens lion*, or *dande lion*.

In China, the whole plant is used. In the United States, the leaves and roots are separated, so you can choose dandelion *leaves* or *root* for your tea.

Dandelion Leaves

Anemia. Dandelion's leaves have iron and vitamin C, which is needed to help iron absorb properly. It's a tea to take for anemia.

Constipation. A mild laxative to relieve constipation and bloating.

Digestion. Dandelion's bitters activate the digestive system, stimulate the flow of natural digestive juices, and prevent indigestion.

Water Retention. Dandelion leaves are a safe and healthy diuretic, because of their potassium content. Most diuretics cause your body to lose potassium, but dandelion leaves restore it. This unique property makes dandelion leaves the herbal remedy for water retention in extremities such as hands, fingers, feet, ankles, calves. Drink your dandelion tea cool or iced.

Weight Control. Good digestion and elimination are important factors for weight control. Dandelion leaves improve both.

Dandelion Root

Detoxifier. Chronic toxic conditions are treated with dandelion root. It removes pesticides, pollutants, contaminants, wastes, and toxins that collect in your joints. In turn, this helps to prevent arthritic inflammations from toxins in joints, and cell damage from free radicals.

A Dandy Winter Tea

A tea of dandelion leaves is a winter cleanser, when heavy food and less activity slow you down. It flushes wastes, recharges digestion, relieves water retention, and has iron and potassium. It's a tea to ring in the new year, after all that holiday eating!

Liver Tonic. A popular liver tonic, dandelion root cools and cleans the liver. It has a long history of use in China and India for all liver complaints, including hepatitis, jaundice, boils, and abscesses.

A Dandy Spring Tonic

Dandelion root is a spring tonic, to cleanse your body of toxins, so you can greet the warm weather with a cool, clean feeling!

Mood Swings. In Chinese medicine, mood swings are associated with too much liver *heat*. Dandelion root cools the liver, and removes toxins to improve everything, including your mood.

Prostate Cleansing. The diuretic and antibacterial

properties in dandelion root have led to its use for prostate infections.

Rheumatism. Dandelion root is antirheumatic.

Urinary Tract. Dandelion root is good for the urinary tract. It's often an ingredient in patent medicines and has been used to dissolve urinary stones.

Uses Through the Ages. In France, blanched young dandelion leaves are used in spring salads. In Britain, the flowers are used for dandelion wine. Dandelion juice is a favorite digestive tonic in domestic medicine. The root has been used to dissolve gallstones, and as an aid in diabetes, since it stimulates the pancreas, which increases insulin production.

Beneficent Parts: Roots and leaves

Properties: Leaves—Potassium, Carotenoids, Bitter Glycosides, Vitamins A, B, C, D, Iron, Choline, Terpenoids; Root—Volatile Oil, Bitter Glycosides, Tannins, Triterpenes, Inulin, Sterols, Choline, Asparagin

Values: Diuretic, Antirheumatic, Laxative, Digestive Tonic, Detoxifier, Liver Cleanser

※

DONG QUAI   *Angelica sinensis*
Also called TANG KUEI
The Supreme Woman's Root

This native of China is a member of the carrot family and a relative of *Angelica archangelica*, an herb that is credited with angelic virtues. The plant has a flowing design that branches out with rich, green, serrated leaves and umbrellalike clusters of tiny white flowers. Its root is brown and fleshy.

Dong quai is a favorite in Chinese blends, and more than two thousand years of use has given it a reputation as *the supreme female tonic*, but it is equally valuable for both sexes. It is a totally wholesome herb with a broad spectrum of health-enriching properties.

"Chi" Energy. Dong quai is a vital energy tonic with high-level nutrition that builds "Chi" energy, to strengthen the vital life force. It is also known as a *dispersing herb*—one that can "move" stagnated body fluids (such as the blood) and redistribute the fluids throughout the body for more balance and harmony in the whole body system. It has a very special ability to penetrate small, thin passageways to remove stagnation.

Digestion. A fine digestive regulator, dong quai eases bloating, soothes stomach cramps, calms the entire digestive tract.

Disease Resistance. Dong quai is antiviral, antifungal, and it fights bacteria. It contains selenium, which helps to build your body's natural barrier to disease, and it has antioxidant vitamin E, for proper absorption of selenium. It also contains silica for tissue repair, iron for healthy blood, and a wealth of other nutrients to strengthen your immunity.

Heart and Blood. It is the most respected heart tonic in the East, because it can dispel patterns of blood stagnation, and that helps to dissolve blood clots. It increases circulation, improves coronary function, and stimulates the production of red blood cells. Its overall effect is soothing, which helps to stabilize minor heart irregularities, and it relaxes the heart muscle to relieve stress on the heart.

Liver. Disperses stagnant energy and clears liver toxins.

Muscles. Dong quai is a restorative tea for muscles and joints. It's antirheumatic and the dried herb or herb from a tea bag can be used externally as a topical compress on the site of an arthritic or rheumatic ache. To make a topical compress, soak a white cotton cloth in hot dong quai tea and apply to the site. It penetrates deep to reduce inflammation, remove toxins, ease aches, and it stimulates circulation to relieve pressure on the site.

Nerves. Dong quai tea carries nutrients for internal tranquillity, including magnesium, B12, and vitamin E. It's also warming.

PMS. Dong quai is a relaxing tea for menses disorders, including PMS tension—it contains zinc and calcium, which are often lacking in women who struggle with PMS depression.

Special Feature: Supreme Woman's Menopause

This is the soundest herb to use for the cycle of hormonal change. It stabilizes estrogen/progesterone production, and it does it without estrogenic properties. It's a powerful source of nutrients to boost vitality. It guards your heart, and helps to build bone marrow which can be a defense against osteoporosis—two very important concerns in menopause. It's a soothing, sweet drink that calms your nervous system and eases internal stress. It stimulates circulation, which enhances concentration and memory. It contains a healthy amount of antiaging vitamin E.

Caution: Avoid dong quai if you have diabetes.

Beneficent Part: Root

Properties: High in Vitamin E; Iron, Vitamins A, B3, B12, B-Complex, C, Calcium, Sodium, Zinc, Magnesium, Phosphorus, Potassium, Selenium, Silicon—Volatile Oil, Bitter Iridoids, Resin, Coumarins, Valerianic Acid, Tannins

Values: Dispersing Herb, Blood Tonic, Antispasmodic, Anti-inflammatory, Antiviral, Antifungal, Digestive Tonic, Antirheumatic, Circulatory Stimulant, Hormone Stabilizer, Mildly Expectorant, Relieves Constipation

ECHINACEA   *Echinacea angustifolia, purpurea, pallida*
Immune System Beauty

This North American perennial is the monarch of the modern-day herb garden. It has dark green leaves, big stems, large flowers with "daisy" petals, and a many-faceted cone center that is radiant in the sun. The plant has deep, medicinal roots, with three varieties that are specific for immunity.

Angustifolia: Called *Black Samson Coneflower*, it has eight-inch leaves, large orchid or violet flowers, and a dark cone center. It's common in the plains states, and was known as *Missouri Snakeroot* by the Sioux, who used it to treat septic disorders, rabies, and snakebites. It removes toxins and fights infections.

Pallida: The *Pale Purple Coneflower* blooms in rosy purple, with drooping flower petals. It was a panacea herb for the plains Indians, used for all ills. It stimulates production of white "killer" cells and regulates red blood cells. It's a lymph system cleanser, tumor-inhibitor, and it's antiallergenic.

Purpurea: The big *Purple Coneflower* can grow to five feet tall and blooms with large reddish purple flowers that can reach four inches in diameter. It was used as a cure-all by the Indians, and is prized in Europe, where it is used as an immune system stimulant.

All Infections and Immunity. Echinacea tea is a standard for infections at onset to stimulate immunity and recovery—colds, flu, viruses, gland swelling, lymph congestion, boils, abscesses, inflammatory conditions, and immunity that is compromised by prolonged illness, surgery, or rounds of antibiotics. The warm water of the tea releases the properties best! A tincture with alcohol doesn't compare.

The standard for taking echinacea is—*one month maximum, one month break*. If your immunity is very weak, and you take echinacea for more than a week, break after one month. Monthly breaks let your body's own immune responses show their new strength. One cup of tea per day is a moderate and effective dose, but many herbalists recommend up to three cups of tea per day for a more potent remedy. When you take three cups of tea per day, it's best to take a break from echinacea after one week, and if you need to resume for another week, scale down your use to one cup per day.

Virtues for Immunity. Echinacea cleans the blood, kidneys, lymph system, and liver, protects healthy cells against decay, fights invaders including bacteria, viruses, fungus, and microbes. It works on a cellular level for defense against disease. It stimulates the production of T-cells, antibodies, and interferon. It's antiallergenic and anti-inflammatory. It has health-building nutrition, including B-complex vitamins, iron for red blood, calcium for strong bones and teeth, selenium for disease resistance, and silica for tissue repair.

Special feature: Topical Echinacea Skin Toner

Documented evidence from Italian scientists shows that polyphenols in echinacea protect the skin from oxidative damage caused by solar radiation. Sun-damaged collagen loses its ability to contract, and that shows up on your face as wrinkles and roughness, or precancerous growths. Antioxidants in echinacea prevent cellular decay and minimize the effects of sun damage.

These findings indicate what many European women have known for a long time—topical echinacea can work wonders on your skin!

How do you get a potent dose of topical echinacea right in your home? Use echinacea tea for a facial toner. It's pure echinacea herb delivered in water, without dyes or additives! Pat it on with a cotton ball and let its healing benefits soak into your skin.

Topical Echinacea Recipe: To make topical echinacea toner from ready-made tea bags, purchase echinacea tea as a *simple*, without other herbs added to make a blend. Look for a tea that uses two or three echinaceas (augustifolia, purpurea, pallida) in one tea. Use two tea bags of echinacea in one cup of water, let the tea steep to a potent brew, and cool. Use a cotton ball to press the echinacea water into your skin. Refrigerate the remaining liquid for repeated use. Make fresh toner every three days. If you use dried herbs, make the toner with two teaspoons of echinacea herb per cup.

It softens hard skin, and penetrates deep to heal "wicked" skin conditions. It's an excellent toner to use before sunbathing.

Beneficent Parts: Root and rhizome

Properties: Good Source of Vitamins and Minerals, including Vitamins A, B-Complex, B3, C, and E. Rich in Iron. Also has Calcium, Magnesium, Manganese, Potassium, Selenium, Silicon, Sodium, Essential Oil, Polyacetylenes, Polysaccharide, Glycoside, Resin, Betaine, Inulin, Sesquiterpene

Values: Immune Stimulant, Alterative, Antimicrobial, Diaphoretic, Antiallergenic, Antiviral, Antifungal, Anti-inflammatory

᠅

ELDER   *Sambuca nigra*
The Herbal Medicine "Chest"

A native of Europe and Britain, elder has thick, branched stems and moss-green, lance-shaped leaves with deep center seams and serrated edges. It blooms with a profusion of small, delicate, creamy-yellow flowers, and bunches of purple-black berries.

Chest Remedy and Upper Respiratory Conditions

1. Hayfever, Allergies. Elder tea clears the upper respiratory tract and removes mucous from the lungs to minimize allergic reactions that can cause hay fever, stuffiness, and tightness in the chest.

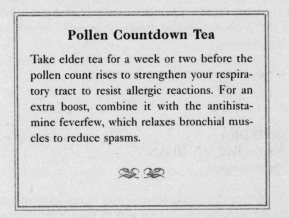

Pollen Countdown Tea

Take elder tea for a week or two before the pollen count rises to strengthen your respiratory tract to resist allergic reactions. For an extra boost, combine it with the antihistamine feverfew, which relaxes bronchial muscles to reduce spasms.

2. Colds, Coughs, and Flu. Elder has a long history as a remedy for colds, coughs, and flu. The hot tea moves imbedded phlegm and helps to clear the respiratory passages. In Israel, elder berries are combined with raspberry and citric acid for a *sambuca* syrup remedy for colds, flu, coughs, and congestion—you can make it as a tea, using elder, raspberry, and lemon. Hot elder berry wine is an old English cold remedy.

Skin (Freckles). Elder water was an 18th century remedy to reduce freckles and whiten the skin. You can use the tea as a skin tonic.

Tonsillitis, Sore Throats. Elder tea is an excellent gargle for throat and mouth infections.

Uses Through the Ages. Elder tea has been used as a children's cold remedy to provide a restful sleep. It also been used for eruptive infections such as measles and chickenpox to cleanse toxins, reduce fevers, and ease inflammation. A half-strength tea is recommended for children's elder tea.

Beneficent Parts: Flowers and Berries

Properties: Volatile Oil, Palmitic, Linoleic, Linolenic Acids, Triterpenes, Flavonoids, Mucilage, Tannins, Pectin, Sugar; Berries Have a High Content of Vitamins A and C, Cyanogenic Glucoside, Viburnic Acid, Alkaloid

Values: Circulatory Stimulant, Expectorant, Phlegm Remedy, Fever Reducer, Diuretic, Topical Anti-inflammatory

∂∂

EPHEDRA   *Ephedra vulgaris, sinica*
Also called MA HUANG
The Stimulant

Native to China, Siberia, and Japan, ephedra can be found on sandy seashores and in temperate climates. It has slender branches with small scaly leaves that join at the base. It produces a succulent cone fruit.

Ephedra contains the alkaloid salt ephedrine, which is the source of the medicine ephedrine, first isolated by Chinese scientists in 1904, and later used in America for the pharmaceutical version. This is a serious medicinal herb with a sympathetic nerve stimulant that resembles adrenaline. Seek professional guidance and your physician's consent before using ephedra.

Asthma. Ephedra has been used for centuries in China as an antiasthmatic, to relieve swelling of the mucous membranes, and ease bronchial spasms in the air passages. *(Try plantain tea instead)*

Colds With Chills. The twigs of ephedra promote

sweating and are used in China for colds and chills. *(Try ginger tea instead)*

Night Sweats. The roots reduce sweating, and are used in China to treat night sweats or chronic sweating conditions. *(Try sage tea instead)*

Caution: Ephedra is not recommended for people taking antidepressants, or for anyone with heart problems, hypertension, or glaucoma.

Beneficent Parts: Twigs and roots

Properties: Volatile Oil, Alkaloids, Saponins

Values: Twigs: Antispasmodic, Fever Reducer, Promotes Sweating, Diuretic, Antibacterial, Antiviral. Roots Reduce Sweating

❧

EUCALYPTUS   *Eucalyptus globulus*
The Big Fever Beater

A native of Australia and Tasmania, the eucalyptus tree has large, leathery leaves dotted with glands that contain a volatile oil called eucalyptol oil. The medicinal tree is known as *The Fever Tree*, because it is a powerful antimicrobial and bacteria fighter wherever it grows. It repels insects and has an antiseptic effect on the air around it.

It was planted in the dreaded fever zone of Algeria to fight malaria, and within five years, the air was healthy to breathe again. It is cultivated in Sicily to prevent malaria. It is one of nature's best cleansers of the environment.

Sickroom Air. Steam from eucalyptus has been used to kill bacteria and microbes to clean the air in sickrooms.

Uses Through the Ages. Eucalyptus has been used as a steam inhalant for chest congestion. Australian settlers used Eucalyptus leaves as a poultice to disinfect blisters and burns.

Caution: Eucalyptus is rarely used internally, but it

can be found in small amounts in blends for coughs, cough syrups, and throat lozenges. Many people say that eucalyptus gives them a feeling of tightness in the chest, and it can affect respiration. A more wholesome herb that is antimicrobial for a respiratory steam inhalant is thyme.

Beneficent Part: Oil from leaves

Properties: Eucalyptol Oil

Values: Purifier

∽

EYEBRIGHT   *Euphrasia officinalis*
The Spirit of Gladness

Native to England, Europe, Asia, and North America, eyebright is a graceful little shrub, no more than eight inches high, found on heaths, moors, and dry pastures. It has a wiry stem and bright green leaves with serrated edges. Among the twenty species of eyebright, the shape of the leaves can vary from pointed and narrow, to round. From July to September, eyebright blooms in clusters of small white or lilac flowers, tinged with yellow. It's one of the few plants that prefers to have grass growing next to it.

Nature has given eyebright real insurance to survive. When a bee visits the flower, pollen falls all over the bee's head, and when he visits the next flower, even if he's just carousing, cross-fertilization occurs as his head bumps into the flower.

Gift from the Graces

Eyebright's official name *Euphrasia* is derived from *Euphrosyne*, Greek meaning "gladness." Euphrosyne was one of the three graces. It is said that she was given the plant to bring to mankind as a medicine to preserve eye-sight.

In the 14th century, it was considered a cure-all for "all evils of the eye" and source of a "precious water to clear a man's spirit."

All of the great herbalists considered eyebright a "specific"—meaning that you use it alone. It has been combined with the herb golden seal, for an eyewash, but it needs no other herb to do its job.

In France, it is known as *casse-lunette*—consolation of the eyes.

It captured the eye of many poets including Milton and Spencer, who called it "Euphrasy." In *Paradise Lost*, Milton told the story of the archangel Michael who doctored Adam after the fall. He wrote:

> *Michael, from Adam's eyes the film removed,*
> *then purged with euphrasine (eyebright) and rue,*
> *his visual orbs, for he had much to see.*

Eyes. For tired, dry eyes; inflamed eyes; eye infections and disorders, try eyebright tea. Bathe your eyes in cool eyebright tea for a very soothing treatment. For chronic cases of eyestrain, bathe eyes three times a day.

Eyes on Computers. Eyebright tea at the office will not only help to prevent those weary computer eyes, it's good for clearing the head, improving memory and sight, and it's mildly tonic.

Eyes, Nose, and Throat. Eyebright acts specifically on the mucous lining of the eyes, nose, and upper throat, to the top of the windpipe to soothe and heal. It can be used regularly as a protective tea to insure health. If you tend to get repeated eye, nose, or throat infections, try eyebright tea for a few weeks to strengthen these areas. It is also a good *safeguard* tea for people who inhale smoke.

Just Plain Grace

Eyebright tea, warm or iced, is soothing, pleasant, and healing to your eyes, nose, throat, and entire windpipe. It helps to clear your head and lift your spirit.

Eyes on Pets. Eye infections and inflammations are common in pets, and they love this soothing eye wash. Treat their eyes to a cool tea eyewash, and use it intermittently to preserve sharp, healthy eyes on your pet.

Hay Fever. Eyebright's astringent properties soothe the mucous lining of the eyes, nose, and throat, and this makes eyebright valuable for hay fever.

Uses Through the Ages. In days of old, eyebright was used for "all infirmities of the eyes." In Russian folk medicine, eyebright was mentioned as a treatment for tired eyes. In Queen Elizabeth's time, an ale was made from eyebright and the dried herb was an ingredient in British Herbal Tobacco, smoked for chronic bronchial colds.

Beneficent Part: The whole plant above the root, when it's flowering

Properties: Good Source of Vitamins and Minerals including Vitamins A, C, D, and E, Calcium, Iodine, Magnesium, Manganese, Silicon, Sodium, Copper and Zinc, Euphrases, Tannin, Mannite, Glucose

Values: Astringent, Mild Tonic, Anti-inflammatory

FENNEL
The Regulator

Foeniculum vulgare

Native to Mediterranean countries, this member of the carrot family also grows wild in Europe and England. Tall and statuesque, the plant has large, glossy stems and light, feathery leaves that alternate on the stem. It blooms in clusters or *umbels* (umbrellalike form) of small yellow flowers that yield small greenish-brown seeds with a licorice flavor.

In Greek myth, according to Sophocles, Prometheus used a hollow stem of fennel to carry fire from heaven for mankind. Fire gave us the ability to cook food, and fennel, which carried the fire, is renowned as a curative plant for digestive disorders.

Digestive Disorders—Indigestion, Heartburn, Gas, Excess Acidity, Constipation, Stomach Discomfort. Fennel is often used in blends for digestive disturbances, since it stimulates the secretion of digestive enzymes, calms the digestive tract, prevents spasms, and improves the absorption of nutrients. It also provides nutrients to restore strength and vigor. To treat digestive disturbances, take one cup of fennel tea after meals until your digestive balance is restored, then use fennel tea as an intermittent toning treatment. It's especially good during the holiday season when heavy eating and poor digestion can throw your system off balance.

Dimmed Vision. Fennel water as an eyewash improves dimmed vision, often perceived as a film over the eyes. Romans believed that snakes got their clear vision from fennel's juice. Fennel water can be made as a mild tea. Let the tea cool and bathe your eyes daily until the condition improves.

Fluid Retention. A natural diuretic, fennel eases bloating and relieves swollen ankles, hands, and hormonal puffiness.

Gums. As a mouth gargle, fennel tea is excellent for gum disorders, laryngitis, and sore throats.

Obesity and Overweight. Fennel has a long tradition of use for weight problems and many old herbals talk about using fennel to achieve slimness.

Fennel "First and Last"

A cup of fennel tea as your first drink in the morning and last drink at night is a time-honored treatment to help to reduce fat.

Strength. Fennel was used by Greek marathon runners for strength, vigor, and leanness. It has a bounty of nutrients to support this use. It contains calcium, magnesium, manganese, phosphorus, sulfur, sodium, silica, iron, selenium, vitamins A, C, and E, and zinc.

Urinary Tract Infections. Fennel has antiseptic volatile oils and diuretic properties which fight infections in the urinary tract and flush out the toxins. It's been used to treat urinary stones and gravel.

Uses Through the Ages. In Chinese medicine, fennel is used to tone the kidneys and spleen, for urinary tract disorders and abdominal pain.

Caution: Moderate use is recommended. Avoid fennel if you are prone to blood clots.

Beneficent Part: Seeds

Properties: Antiseptic Volatile Oils, Essential Fatty Acids, Flavonoids (Rutin), High in Nutrients

Values: Circulatory Tonic, Eases Cramps and Spasms, Stimulant, Anti-inflammatory, Diuretic, Mild Expectorant, Estrogenic Effect

☙

FENUGREEK
The Tummy Tamer

Trigonella-foenum-graecum

A native of North Africa and India, fenugreek has long, slim stems; bright green leaves; light yellow flowers; and brownish-yellow seeds.

Stomach Upsets, Indigestion. Fenugreek has a long history of use for stomach troubles. In China it is used for abdominal pain. In Egypt, it's a standard tea for tourists with stomach upsets. A warm, comforting brew for the stomach, fenugreek is anti-inflammatory, cleansing, and has a soothing mucilage that coats and moisturizes an aggravated stomach lining. The mild maple flavor of fenugreek peaks with a little honey and lemon.

Uses Through the Ages. Fenugreek has been used for sinus and ear congestion, as an aid in non-insulin-dependent diabetes since it lowers blood sugar levels.

Special Feature: Natural plant protein

Fenugreek has protein and protein-digesting enzymes for vegetarians, muscle builders, and fatigued people who may not be digesting and assimilating their proteins.

Beneficent Part: Seeds

Properties: Protein—Including Tryptophan, Vitamins A, B-Complex, C, D, Calcium, Iron, Lysine, Magnesium, Phosphorus, Potassium, Selenium, Sodium, Zinc—Alkaloids, Mucilage, Estrogenlike Steroidal Saponins

Values: Anti-inflammatory, Aphrodisiac, Demulcent, Digestive Tonic, Uterine Stimulant

☙

FEVERFEW
Chrysanthemum parthenium
Manna for Migraines and Allergies
Tanacetum parthenium

A native of Europe and Britain and member of the daisy family, feverfew is a hardy plant with hairy stems, many branches, and downy leaves that can be hairy or smooth. It blooms with small, yellow, daisylike flowers.

Allergies, Asthma, Hay Fever. Feverfew is a natural antihistamine to combat allergic reactions and hay fever. Hot feverfew tea relieves the symptoms of asthma, allergies, and hay fever by inhibiting the release of histamines which are linked to allergic reactions. It clears phlegm, decongests the chest and sinuses, and relaxes tension to relieve bronchial spasms.

Digestive Remedy. Feverfew has bitters to calm and strengthen the digestive tract. It stimulates the liver, which aids in the production of digestive enzymes, and it clears heat from the body to ease indigestion.

Headaches, Migraines. Studies indicate that feverfew can help to prevent headaches and migraines when it is taken as a routine health treatment. Headaches have been associated with histamines in the body, and feverfew inhibits histamine release. It also relaxes blood vessels and is a tonic for the nerves to relieve tension headaches. In addition, feverfew is a liver stimulant, and liver weakness is associated with headaches. Feverfew tea can be taken during a headache to help to relieve tension, but its best use is as a regular health treatment for people who suffer with recurring headaches or migraines, to help to prevent their recurrence.

PMS. Feverfew tea can be used for premenstrual headaches, tension, and periods that are slow to start. Feverfew is a uterine stimulant that also has a relaxing effect. This makes it an ideal remedy to ease the pent-up feelings of PMS. It helps to initiate blood flow in "clogged" or delayed periods. It also stimulates the liver,

Migraine Recipe

Warm feverfew tea taken twice a day is the recommended treatment to speed your recovery from a migraine. For a follow-up treatment after a migraine, take feverfew tea once a day for a week.

which helps to relieve irritability and headaches, which are often related to sluggish livers.

Uses Through the Ages. Feverfew was used in England as an anti-inflammatory for arthritic conditions. It has also been used to calm the nerves for sciatica and neuralgia.

Caution: Avoid feverfew if you take blood-thinning medication.

Beneficent Parts: Leaves, flowers, stems

Properties: Vitamins and Minerals, including A, C, B-Complex, Iron, Potassium, Magnesium, Manganese, Selenium, Sodium, Zinc, Volatile Oil, Pyrethrin, Tannins, Sesquiterpene Lactones, Bitter Resin

Values: Anti-inflammatory, Relaxes Blood Vessels, Uterine Stimulant, Digestive Stimulant, Brings on Menstruation, Expels Worms

FLAX
More Than a Laxative

Linum catharticum
Linum usitatissimum

Flax's seeds have been revered as a health *food* for centuries. They were used by the Greeks, mandated by law as a necessary food in the 8th century in France, and recommended by Gandhi. The oil from flax is the well-known linseed oil, an important source of essential fatty acids. The tea from flax is traditionally made from the whole plant, and since it is a bulking laxative, it is often found in blends for intestinal cleansing and rheumatism. A tea can be made from flax seeds, and they have a special contribution to make to health.

Cystitis. Flax seed tea is soothing and cleansing to the urinary tract and it makes a comforting remedy for cystitis.

Phytochemical Lignans. Flax seeds are one of the richest sources of phytochemical lignans, which have been shown to have anticancer value, and may help to reduce the risks of breast, colon, and prostate cancer. Flax seed tea can be made by crushing the seeds and steeping them in boiling water.

Beneficent Parts: Whole plant, seeds

Properties: Omega-3 Essential Fatty Acids, Linolenic Acid, Linoleic Acid, Proteins, Minerals, Fiber, Calcium, Potassium, Mucilage, Cyanogenic Glycosides

Values: Laxative, Demulcent, Antirheumatic, Health Tonic

❧

GINGER
The Hot Root
Zingiber officinalis

Ginger has been a renowned root for more than two thousand years. When you take it as a tea, it warms you from head to toe. Some say they can feel their legs tingling with renewed circulation.

Arthritis, Rheumatism, Osteoporosis, Gout. Ginger warms and comforts the body, increases blood flow to cleanse toxins and promote healing. It has a good reputation as a remedy for arthritis, rheumatism, osteoporosis, and gout.

Cold and Chills, Cold Hands and Feet. Ginger is a warming tea that is also a mild expectorant, which is very beneficial for cold conditions, including colds, chills, and congestion. It's a fine tea to take when you feel cold, lack an appetite, or have cold hands and feet.

Heart Health. Ginger is a gem for the heart. It lowers cholesterol, stabilizes blood pressure and heart functions, helps to prevent clotting, and reduces the risk of heart attacks and strokes.

Nausea, Motion Sickness. Ginger stops nausea and queasiness better than any pill. A cup of ginger tea before you travel will calm you all over.

Weight Control and Digestion. Ginger stimulates saliva, digestive enzymes for proteins and fats, and it increases metabolic heat to burn calories.

Uses Through the Ages. In the 18th century, ginger was used in blends to balance other herbs and soothe the stomach. In China, it is used for colds and chills, and it's considered a "yang" tonic for spleen energy.

Caution: Use moderately. Avoid ginger if you have peptic ulcers.

Beneficent Part: Root

Properties: Alkaloids, Mucilage, Phenols, Volatile Oil

Values: Antispasmodic, Antiseptic, Carminative, Circulatory Stimulant, Expectorant, Tonic

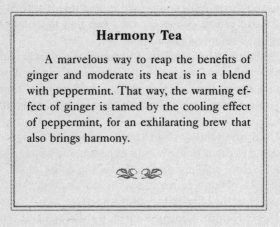

Harmony Tea

A marvelous way to reap the benefits of ginger and moderate its heat is in a blend with peppermint. That way, the warming effect of ginger is tamed by the cooling effect of peppermint, for an exhilarating brew that also brings harmony.

GINKGO   *Ginkgo biloba*
The Life Enhancer

Ginkgo is a 200-million-year-old tree from the age of the dinosaurs and the oldest living tree. It's known for its odd scent, double-lobed leaves, and small round fruits that ripen to an apricot color. The name *ginkgo* comes from the Chinese *Yin Guo* or *hill apricot*, for the color of its fruit, and *biloba* for the double lobes of its leaves. It was the lone survivor of the atomic blast in Hiroshima. Today, ginkgo trees are commonly found in cities, where they thrive despite pollution, bacteria, viruses, and insects.

The leaves of this enduring tree have some remark-

able properties that provide healthy endurance for
people.

Allergies, Asthma. An allergic substance called PAF
has been found to be more prevalent in people with
asthma and allergies, and it is believed that PAF contrib-
utes to allergic reactions. Ginkgo helps to block the production of PAF, which makes it a valuable tea for people
with asthma and allergies. In China, a tea of ginkgo is
used as a throat spray, and studies show that allergic reactions are noticeably reduced by the spray. To make a
throat spray with ginkgo tea, sterilize a spray bottle by
boiling it, and prepare two bags of ginkgo tea in one cup
of water. Keep your spray bottle in the refrigerator to be
within reach for allergic reactions. Also, you can gargle
with ginkgo tea to combat an allergic reaction.

Circulation. Blood circulation is the source of nourishment for every process in your body from the smallest
cells, capillaries, arteries, and veins, to bones, muscles,
organs, and the largest organ—your skin. When your circulation is blocked or hampered in its flow, it can lead to
many premature health disturbances including premature aging of cells, atrophy in veins and extremities—
which lead to varicose veins, leg pains, joint aches, and
difficulty in walking. In addition, insufficient blood flow
to the brain reduces your ability to concentrate, and can
lead to depression, poor memory, balance problems, vision problems, headaches, and stroke. Ginkgo is one of
the most respected herbs for circulation problems. Its
ginkgolides stimulate circulation to the brain and extremities, which prevent many symptoms of aging, including memory loss, disorientation, hearing disorders,
and strokes. A three-month study of gingko's effect on
golden-age people showed that ginkgo relieved symptoms of disorientation, memory loss, anxiety, tinnitus, and
headaches in 92 percent of the test subjects. It is cur-

rently being studied for its ability to reduce these symptoms in Alzheimer's patients.

Tree of Life Tea

A cup of ginkgo tea is a healthy daily
habit to keep you at your peak of fitness. It's
the ideal tea to counteract the effects of sedentary work days and it helps to keep you
youthful as you age.

❧ ❧

Heart. Ginkgo's value as a circulatory tonic is also
vital for a healthy heart, to prevent high blood pressure.
Its antioxidants are free radical scavengers, which help to
keep heart passages free of deposits. Research indicates
that ginkgo can treat irregular heartbeat, without side effects.

Stroke. Strokes often occur when blood supply to the
brain is weak or hampered. It is the second most common cause of death in the United States. By improving
circulation, ginkgo enables your brain to get more oxygen
and glucose, the fuel it needs for healthy maintenance.
Ginkgo also has been shown to have a soothing effect on
arteries, which can prevent spasms in brain arteries,
which can also lead to strokes.

Uses Through the Ages. Ginkgo is used in China for
asthma, congestion, lung weakness, hearing disorders,
and longevity. In traditional Chinese medicine, ginkgo is
used in combination with other herbs in order to enhance
the healing value of the blend.

Beneficent Parts: Leaves and seeds

Properties: Leaves—Flavonoid Ginkosides, Quercetin, Proanthocy-anidins, Lactones, Terpenes, Sito-sterol; Seeds—Bioflavones, Minerals, Fatty Acids

Values: Leaves—Nervine, Stimulant, Astringent, Diaphoretic; Seeds—Astringent, Antifungal, Antibacterial

♉

GINSENG Chinese, Korean, Asian: *Panax Ginseng,* American: *Panax Quinquefolius*

The King of Tonics   Siberian: *Eleutherococcus senticoccus acanthopanax*

Indigenous to China, Manchuria, eastern Asia, North America, and cultivated in Korea and Japan, ginseng is a perennial plant that proclaims *balance* in its form. It has a simple stem, with leaves forming opposites on the stem, each leaf divided into five leaflets with serrated edges. It has small yellow flowers that also bloom in opposites, with a crown of one top bloom, followed by clusters of bright red berries.

Ginseng's root grows slowly, often taking three years to reach maturity. It is spindle shaped, fleshy, and ringed, with colors ranging from light yellow to brown.

The Man Root

Ginseng has been known by many names, including *five fingers* for its five leaflets, *red berry* for its berries, and *man's health* or *man root* by the Chinese, who see a man's body in the root's form. It was used by Arab physicians in the 9th century, and became a popular tonic for wealthy Europeans after Louis XIV received it as a gift from the King of Siam. The name *panax* comes from the Greek *panakos*, meaning "panacea," and *ginseng*, which means "wonder of the world."

A fascinating correlation occurred on opposite sides of the world with ginseng. In China, the panax root was called *Jin Chen*—"like a man," while early American Indians named the American panax root *garantoquen*, which has the same meaning.

Ginseng is so important in China that traditionally only the emperor could collect the roots. In America, the best roots were the light-colored ones collected by Sioux women, who cleaned the roots by rotating them in water in a barrel, with rods running lengthwise to turn the roots.

The root's appearance gives ginseng its value, and connoisseurs look for the largest size, lightest color, the plumpest and most unbroken—closest to its natural form.

White ginseng is cool, recommended for summer.
Red ginseng is warm, recommended for winter.

The Root with Many Uses

While the different varieties can have their own unique values, in general there are many virtues attributed to the King of Tonics. Ginseng is an *adaptogen*—an herb that balances opposites and helps the body defend itself from stress. For centuries, it has been used to strengthen organs, calm nerves, stop heart palpitations, brighten vision, increase mental ability, and provide a youthful feeling. Many Asians feel that ginseng is wasted on the young, and is best for advanced age, to increase energy, sexual vigor, muscle tone, skin tone, resistance to stress, and to enhance immunity.

It is generally agreed that ginseng is a powerful antidote to stress, debility, weakness, and problems of aging. It acts on the pituitary and adrenal glands and stimulates the nervous system to decrease fatigue. It has a solid nutrient content that provides a strong base for its invigorating values.

Ginseng has antioxidants to prevent cellular aging. It raises HDL (good cholesterol), helps to regulate blood sugar levels, deep-cleans the tissues, and stimulates the production of red and white blood cells for better defense against disease. It increases hormone secretions in the endocrine system and can be a tonic for the libido, to fight impotence and frigidity. It is especially useful to fight exhaustion and depression that stem from nervous disorders.

It is also generally agreed that regular use (six months) is needed to see these results, but many herbalists don't recommend taking ginseng for more than a month.

In China, small amounts of ginseng are common in most remedies, and it has been used to ward off disease and degeneration for five thousand years. The root is chewed to increase vitality, recover from debility, treat lung disorders, dissolve tumors, and prolong life.

Large doses of ginseng are not better than small, steady doses. It's a tonic herb, and consistency counts more than bursts of potency. The easiest and least costly way to get steady, consistent doses of ginseng is by taking ginseng as a tea.

Caution: Ginseng is a tonic that should be avoided if you have inflammatory conditions, bronchitis, high blood pressure, or if you take other stimulants.

Beneficent Part: Root, collected in August to retain plumpness

Properties: Saponins (Hormone Like Ginsenosides), Volatile Oil, Sterols, Starch, Pectin, Resin, Vitamins B1, B2, B12, D, Fats, Iron, Calcium, Manganese, Vanadium, Magnesium, Copper, Zinc, Antioxidant

Values: Antidepressant, Tonic, Adaptogen, Aphrodisiac, Nervine,

Stimulates Immune System, Regulates Blood Sugar and Cholesterol
Levels

❧

GOLDENSEAL   *Hydrastis canadensis*
The Rare Root

A North American treasure that grows wild in woody
areas of Canada and the eastern United States, golden
seal is a member of the buttercup family that is known
for its odd appearance. It has a hairy stem with hairs that
point down, dark green wrinkled leaves that are also
hairy. It produces an inedible crimson berry and skimpy
greenish flowers.

Early Indian medicine men found goldenseal's
beauty underground. Horizontal, knotted, and irregular,
the bright yellow root of goldenseal is big medicine.

A Proud Tradition

Goldenseal was a favorite of the Cherokee Indians,
and was called "the Cherokee cure for cancer." They
used it to heal local inflammations and digestive disorders. The Iroquois used it for whooping cough, liver disorders, heart problems, and fevers. It's been called by
many names, including *Yellow Root, Orange Root, Turmeric
Root, Eye Root, Eye Balm, Indian Paint, Indian Dye,* and
even *Ground Raspberry,* from its raspberrylike leaves and
red fruit. The first settlers learned the virtues of goldenseal from the American Indian natives who used the root
for their medicine, and the yellow juice for fabric dye
and face paint.

Its name comes from seallike markings on its root,
which retains the scars from the former years' stems.

Goldenseal is one of the herbs that literally gives up

its life for its use as medicine. It takes three years for the root to mature for medicinal value, and in the fourth year, the root begins to die. Propagating new plants is difficult, making goldenseal one of the rarest herbs. For lovers of herbs and herbal remedies, a box of goldenseal tea is a treasure to use with respect. Think of goldenseal for its external uses first! For internal issues, use it sparingly.

Eye Balm. Goldenseal tea is an antibiotic and astringent water that is beneficial for eye inflammations. It has been used for pink eye, conjunctivitis, and all eye infections. Use the tea to bathe your eyes, or you can use warm tea bags to cover your eyes for a treatment.

Golden Gargle. A powerful medicine to use for gum infections, mouth sores, and sore throats, goldenseal dries and disinfects swollen, aggravated tissues, and keeps infections from spreading. Use the tea for your gargle.

Mucous Membranes. Goldenseal is a renowned tonic and disinfectant for the mucous membranes of your body. From head to toe, it reduces inflammation, clears phlegm, and has strong antiviral and antibacterial action to combat the infections that inflame the mucous lining. If you are congested with phlegm, as can happen with a particularly brutal cold, goldenseal can dry out the mucous quickly, inhibit the spread of bacteria, and virtually calm you as you drink it. It's especially attuned to upper respiratory infections, and a real go-getter for unhealthy intestinal bacteria.

Vaginal Infections. This is a four-star treatment! Goldenseal tea can be used for a vaginal douche to treat those hard-to-reach tissues to a bath of relief, to combat discharges and yeast infections. Pour your goldenseal tea into a standard douche holder and top it off with water. Use during and after an infection to insure that the tissues are thoroughly cleansed. It's also an excellent treatment to use every few months for maintenance.

Wounds. One of the best wound cleansers and healers, goldenseal knocks off bacteria, coats the tissues to inhibit infections, heals, and seals. To give you an idea of the extent of wounds it heals, the Cherokees used it to fill the holes of bullet wounds for swift return to battle. Use goldenseal tea on any wound or skin condition including eczema, seborrhea, impetigo, cuts, rashes, ulcers, ringworm, persistent bacterial infections, and as a wash for measles.

Uses Through the Ages. Goldenseal has been used to treat menses disorders, especially heavy bleeding, and menopausal transitions, since it reduces sweating. It has been a treatment for digestive disorders, liver disorders, lupus, hay fever, hemorrhoids, poor circulation, and all stomach infections. It's been called a spinal nerve tonic, and was used to fight meningitis. Also, it has a tradition of use for sexually transmitted diseases. It's a natural substitute for quinine.

Caution: Goldenseal is an herb to use very prudently for internal problems. You don't need a lot to accomplish results. One cup of goldenseal tea, sipped slowly, will give you substantial relief from mucous buildup during chronic colds for phlegm, chest congestion, or a flare-up of spastic colon or colitis. Goldenseal shouldn't be taken for more than 8–10 days, and even then, it would be best to take it every other day. It's very drying and medicinal, and for this reason, it's often used in small amounts in herbal blends.

Very high doses of goldenseal can cause toxicity. Not recommended for people with heart problems, high blood pressure, diabetes, glaucoma, history of stroke, or hypoglycemia. While one of its ingredients, berberine, lowers blood pressure, another ingredient, hydrastin, raises it.

Beneficent Parts: Root and rhizome

Properties: Vitamins A, B-Complex, C, Calcium, Phosphorus, Potassium, Magnesium, Selenium, Zinc, Iron, Manganese, Silicon, Alkaloids Berberine, Hydrastine, Canadine, Resin, Volatile Oil, Bitters

Values: Circulatory Tonic, Digestive Tonic, Mucous Cleanser, Alterative, Laxative, Stomachic, Astringent, Antibiotic, Antiviral, Antimicrobial

☙

GOTU KOLA   *Centella asiatica*
Sanskrit Name: MADOOKAPARNI
The Herb for the Brain

A native of Ceylon and revered Ayurvedic herb, gotu kola is a slender, trailing plant that grows anywhere without any particular fuss. It's a plant that's loved by elephants, who are known for their longevity and ability to remember.

Brain Food—Memory, Learning Ability, Concentration. Gotu kola is known as a tonic for the brain. It cleanses the blood, stimulates the central nervous system, improves circulation and oxygen uptake by the brain, inspires clear thinking, better focus, and concentration.

Learning Impaired. In Indian studies on retarded children, those taking gotu kola showed an increase in their IQ on standardized tests and more outgoing behavior skills.

Hormone Balance. Gotu kola is known as "the secret of perpetual youth" for its ability to balance hormones. It stimulates the pituitary gland and thyroid.

Beneficent Part: Herb

Properties: Vitamins A, B-Complex, B2, C, K, Iron, Riboflavin, Magnesium, Manganese, Phosphorus, Sodium, Silicon, Zinc

Values: Circulatory Stimulant, Thyroid Stimulant, Nervine, Tonic,
Diuretic, Mild Laxative

❦

GREEN, OOLONG, BLACK   *Camellia sinensis*
The Legendary Teas

A native of China and one of the oldest medicinal
herbs, *camellia sinensis* is a tall evergreen shrub that
blooms with white flowers that resemble dogwood roses.
This is the shrub that started the legend of tea in 2737
B.C. when the fresh leaves fell into the boiling water of
Chinese Emperor Shen Nung, the father of Chinese
medicine. Today, there are more than three thousand
species of the shrub that yield hundreds—if not thousands—of varieties of the most popular teas in the
world—green, oolong, and black. Green tea comes from
the fresh leaves; oolong from leaves that are mildly fermented; and black, the most pungent of the teas, comes
from fully fermented leaves.

While all three teas can come from the same shrub,
countries specialize in the production of green, oolong, or
black. China produces all three, Japan specializes in
green—which is known as its national beverage. India
takes pride in its black assam teas.

The primary properties of tea leaves are polyphenols,
commonly called *tannins*, which yield the color, strength,
body, and taste that is present in a tea after it is pro-
cessed. In the art of fermenting, the leaves are piled and
sweated, which oxidizes the leaves, darkens their color,
and changes the flavor and aroma. While the fermenta-
tion yields some of the world's most flavorful teas, it
changes the medicinal character. It is believed that the
more fermented the leaves, the weaker the medicinal
nature. Therefore, green is the strongest medicinally,

mildly fermented oolong is second in medicinal strength, and black, the most fermented of the teas, is third.

Green tea is a yellow-green liquor made from the fresh, unfermented, dried leaves, which are usually the top two leaves and bud.

Health and Immunity. Green tea's polyphenols are powerful antioxidants that are reputed to be two hundred times stronger than vitamin E. It has anticancer catekins, which protect the cells from carcinogens, toxins, free radical damage, and help to keep radioactive strontium 90 out of the bones. The catekins are also antibacterial, lower cholesterol, and help to metabolize fats. It reduces blood pressure, helps to regulate blood sugar, and it's a heart stimulant that helps to prevent cardiovascular disease. It's antiviral to fight colds, flu, and viruses.

Healthy Teeth and Gums. Green tea is high in fluoride for healthy teeth, and has compounds that prevent tooth decay and fight gum disease.

Respiratory Problems. Green tea is a bronchial dilator and mild decongestant for respiratory problems, asthma, and breathing difficulties. It can help you to breathe easier.

Stimulant. Green tea is a stimulant with 40–50 milligrams of caffeine in each cup (half the caffeine of coffee). It is often used by Zen monks for hours of wakeful meditation.

In the Japanese tea ceremony, a green tea called *matcha* is made from dried young leaves that have been ground to a fine green powder. One teaspoon of the powder is placed in a tea cup, boiling water is added to the powder, and the brew is whipped with a bamboo whisk.

Since the green teas are very delicate in flavor, water just under a boil is often recommended to preserve the delicacy. Jasmine tea is a green tea with jasmine blossoms.

❧

GUELDER ROSE (see CRAMP BARK)

❧

HAWTHORN
The Heart Herb

Cratagus oxyacantha
Cratagus monogyna

Common to Europe, North Africa, and Western Asia, hawthorn is a bushy member of the rose family with sweet green deep-cut leaves, reddish brown branches, clusters of delicate white flowers, and brilliant purple-red mealy berries (haws). It can reach thirty feet in height and is used for hedges.

Hawthorn has had many names that reveal its characteristics. It blooms in May and was called *May Blossom*. It's growth is rapid, giving it the name *Quick*. It's been called *Whitethorn* for its thorns, *Haw* for its mealy berries, *Hedgethorn* for its use as a hedge.

Since Biblical times, hawthorn has been a "sacred" herb, identified as the bush that was used to make the crown of thorns for Jesus. In Ancient Rome, hawthorn was considered to have magical properties, while in Greece, it was seen as a symbol for hope and joy.

Heart Health. Hawthorn is a heart tonic that opens the arteries and enhances blood circulation through the body. That, in turn, improves uptake of oxygen, helps to regulate heart rate and stabilize blood pressure. Hawthorn is also a *relaxant*—it relieves stress on the nervous system, and it has a diuretic effect to prevent fluid retention—two big factors in heart health. It has been used to ease palpitations, treat irregular pulse and hypertension.

Circulation to the Legs. Sedentary days in our computer age lead to poor circulation in the legs. Hawthorn is the tea to use for legs that get pins and needles, or go "dead," when you sit too long. It's a good tea for older people who need more blood circulation to the extremities. In Chinese medicine, hawthorn berries are called *Shan Zha*, and are used to "move blood."

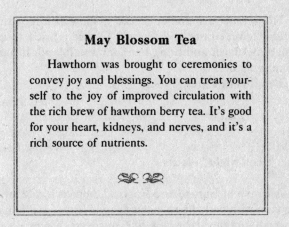

May Blossom Tea

Hawthorn was brought to ceremonies to convey joy and blessings. You can treat yourself to the joy of improved circulation with the rich brew of hawthorn berry tea. It's good for your heart, kidneys, and nerves, and it's a rich source of nutrients.

Memory and Alertness. Hawthorn improves the blood supply to the brain, which clears the cobwebs away, improves your memory and ability to concentrate.

Beneficent Parts: Leaves, flowers, berries

Properties: Vitamins C, A, B-Complex, Sodium, Silicon, Iron, Manganese, Magnesium, Potassium, Phosphorous, Selenium—Saponins, Glycosides, Flavonoids, Tannin, Procyanidines, Trimethylamine

Values: Cardiovascular Tonic, Hypotensive, Vasodilator, Relaxant, Astringent, Antispasmodic, Diuretic

❧

HIBISCUS
An Enhancer for Blends

Hibiscus is a member of the mallow family with a
mellow, sweet taste and vitamin C that is used to enhance the flavor and bring harmony to a blend. It has a
calming nature.
Beneficent Part: Flowers

❧

HOPS   *Humulus lupulus*
The "Good Night" Flowers

A native of Europe and England, hops is a wild twining vine with dark green, heart-shaped leaves and female
flowers (strobiles) that look like small green pine cones.
It's best known for its use in brewing beer, as far back as
the 14th century in the Netherlands. Hops wasn't added
to British beer until the 16th century—its cultivation was
banned in England during the reign of Henry VI, when it
was called an "unwholesome weed." Unwholesome it is
not; since it has a strong vitamin and mineral content, it's
antibiotic, antiseptic, antimicrobial, antispasmodic to relieve tension, and it has bitters to aid digestion.

Hops for Her. Hops is a standard remedy for
women's tension, PMS, and menopause symptoms including anxiety and insomnia, since it contains natural
estrogens in a sedative formula. It's been used for irritable bowel syndrome, diverticulitis, mucous colitis, digestive stress, ulcers, and nervous disorders including
hysteria. It has asparagin to reduce fluid retention, it's a
liver stimulant and blood cleanser, and it has had its
share of praise as an herb to use for healthy, clear skin.

Hops tea used as a steam inhalant is good for throat and chest problems.

But Not for Him. For men, the sedative effect of hops and its estrogenic action is depressing to the libido, and that might be what King Henry found displeasing.

Insomnia. Hops is often used in nighttime tea blends to induce a restful sleep. The Meskwaki Indians used hops to stuff pillows as a sleep aid, and sedative hops pillows are still used today. If you have pollen-sensitive skin, hops pillows could give you a rash.

Beneficent Part: Flowers

Properties: Vitamins A, B-Complex, B3, Potassium, Phosphorus, Calcium, Magnesium, Manganese, Selenium, Silicon, Sodium, Iron, Zinc, Copper, Iodine, Fluorine, Chlorine—Volatile Oil, Bitter Resins, Tannins, Estrogenic Substances, Asparagin

Values: Sedative to Higher Nerve Centers, Antispasmodic, Antimicrobial, Digestive Aid, Antiseptic, Astringent, Diuretic, Pain Reliever, Kills Worms, Reduces Fevers

❧

HOREHOUND, WHITE   *Marrubium vulgare*
The Expectorant

This European member of the mint family is native to Britain, and grows wild in wastelands and by roadsides throughout Europe, although it is rare. It's a bushy herb with branching stems and wrinkled leaves covered with dense white hairs, giving horehound a soft, woolly appearance. The fresh leaves have a musk scent and it blooms with clusters of tiny white flowers.

It was given a place of honor by Egyptian priests, who called horehound *Eye of the Star, Bull's Blood,* and *The Seed of Horus.* It was esteemed as an herb that could dispel magic, in a time when sudden illnesses were often viewed as "magic spells." In Rome it was a medicine, used as an antidote for poisons, snakebites, and rabies. In old England, it was brewed into Horehound Ale, taken as a health beverage.

Expectorant for the Lungs. A popular expectorant, horehound is a pectoral remedy to remove imbedded phlegm. The tea is a treatment for lung problems, asthmatic phlegm, breathing difficulties caused by phlegm, old nagging coughs, phlegm colds, wheezing, and shortness of breath. Horehound tea can be taken in half-cup doses every few hours as an expectorant tonic.

Uses Through the Ages. Horehound has been used to treat uterine fibroids.

Beneficent Parts: Leaves and flowers

Properties: Vitamins A, B-Complex, C, E, Iron, Potassium, Bitter Principle Marrubium, Volatile Oil, Resin, Tannin, Fat, Sugar, Wax

Values: Expectorant, Deobstruent, Tonic, Diaphoretic, Diuretic, Stomachic, Resolvent, Kills Worms

୨୬

HORSETAIL   *Equisetum arvense*
Healing Stems

The plainest of the plain herbs, today's horsetail is a shiny grass, but in prehistoric times, it grew as big as trees. The most interesting feature about horsetail is that it has no leaves, only threadlike, jointed stems or branches that form sharp angles, and end in a razorlike point. They are virtually colorless and tasteless.

According to myth, if you find horsetails growing in a field, it means there is underground water or a spring below. Called *Shave-grass, Bottlebrush, Paddock-pipes, Dutch rushes,* and *Oaks* in Australia, these barren fronds can point to the sky with pride. They are one of the richest sources of silica for tissue repair. The herbalist

Culpepper wrote that horsetail stems can "heal sinews though they be cut asunder."

Tissue Repair. The high concentration of silica in horsetail is manna for internal or external wounds. Taken as a tea for an internal injury, horsetail will stop bleeding and help to repair the tissue in a wound. This makes horsetail tea helpful for bleeding ulcers, cystic ulcers, hemorrhoids, and heavy bleeding in menses. It's an excellent tea to take if you are hemorrhaging and waiting for an ambulance. For an external wound, a bandage soaked in horsetail tea water will work effectively to stop bleeding and start wound healing.

Nosebleeds. Horsetail tea stops nosebleeds. In a nosebleed crisis, to reduce your panic, you can soak a fresh cloth in horsetail tea water, or use the warm tea bag as a compress on the nostril. Drip the horsetail tea water into the nostril if you can. Take the tea internally while you call 911.

Hair, Skin, and Nails. Horsetail tea is rich in silica and calcium to strengthen brittle nails; give life to dull, dry hair; and restore skin tissues. Vitamin combinations for hair, skin, and nails often contain silicon—or the natural silica from horsetails. It's a good tea for postmenopausal women to keep their hair, skin, and nails in fit shape.

Lung Weakness. The silica in horsetails is essential for healthy lung tissues and tissue repair. It was an old-time remedy for all lung disorders and respiratory problems.

Kidney Health. Horsetail is a kidney tonic and has been used for kidney disorders including dropsy, gravel, kidney inflammation, and stones. To swing into spring with healthy kidneys, which help to boost your immunity, try a toning week with horsetail tea.

Prostate and Urinary Tract. Horsetail is attuned to the urinary tract where it reduces inflammation, heals infections, and has mild diuretic properties to remove toxins. At the first sign of urinary discomfort, burning or tingling, horsetail tea can save the day, even keep an infection away. It has been used to treat painful urination, incontinence, and bed-wetting in children, and to cleanse the prostate, helping to prevent enlargement.

Eyelid Swelling. Warm horsetail tea bags on your eyes will reduce puffiness and swelling, while it treats your eyes to a healing silica bath. In Chinese medicine, horsetail is used for eye disorders, including conjunctivitis and corneal distortions.

Bleeding Gums. Horsetail tea used as a gargle to stop bleeding in gums and help to repair the tissues.

Special Feature: That Special Magnetism

In Ayurvedic medicine, silicon is valued for its ability to impart "magnetism" to the nerves. The silica in horsetail is the naturally occurring form of silicon, to nourish your nerves, brain cells, eyes, hair, nails, teeth, skin, and all internal body tissues. Ayurvedic tradition says that lack of silica can make you feel irritable, edgy, and lackluster. When you are rich in silica, you sparkle, radiate energy, and have better body harmony.

Beneficent Part: Stems

Properties: Rich Source of Silica and Calcium, Vitamins A, B1, B2, B3, B5, C, E, Selenium, Magnesium, Potassium, Phosphorus, Iron, Manganese, Sodium, Chlorine, Zinc, Cobalt, Gold, Silver, Platinum, Rhodium—Alkaloids (including Nicotine), Saponins, Tannins, Flavonoids, Phytosterols

Values: Wound Healer, Astringent, Diuretic, Styptic, Tonic

HUANG QI (see ASTRAGALUS)

HYSSOP
Hyssopus officinalis
The Breath of Life

This native of southern Europe is a bushy evergreen with square stems; slim, linear leaves; and whorls of blue flowers.

Its name comes from the Greek *azob,* which means "holy herb." It's one of the herbs that grows on the hills of Palestine, and was traditionally used to clean holy places.

Respiratory System Cleanser. A purgative for the chest and expectorant for stubborn phlegm, hyssop tea is an excellent treatment to maintain the health of your respiratory system, and to strengthen the mucous membranes throughout your body, since it reduces inflammation in the membranes. Mucous congestion and inflammation of the membranes allow bacteria to thrive, and that can compromise your immunity, making you more susceptible to mucous-related disorders, including:

1. Asthmatic "Attacks" and Allergic Reactions. Try hyssop tea as a cleansing remedy when you are not in the spell of an "attack" or "reaction." That way, you will reap the benefits of hyssop's expectorant action as a *health treatment.* The renowned herbalist E. M. Grieves wrote that hyssop tea "admirably promotes expectoration." It has no known toxicity, and is totally safe to use more often if you need it. As you continue with the treatment, one day you might see that your attacks or allergic reactions don't seem to occur as frequently. Then you're on your way to real relief. When mucous congestion is relieved, it makes the "Breath of Life" go that much deeper.

2. Bronchitis, or Lingering Bronchial Congestion. Hyssop tea helps to purge bronchial mucous and cleanse bronchial passages.

3. Congested Chest Colds. If you feel "all choked up" with a cold, try this treatment. Take plantain tea to dry the mucous and help you breathe—it can clear a congested chest in twenty minutes or less. Afterward, try a cleansing treatment of hyssop tea to bring up imbedded mucous, to insure that bacteria doesn't stay behind in your mucous membranes. Hyssop can be combined with horehound for chronic chest congestion.

4. Breathing Difficulties, Wheezing. Use a treatment of hyssop tea to expectorate mucous plugs and to help you breathe more deeply. Stay with it until you gain more respiratory strength.

Rheumatism. Hyssop tea is a traditional remedy for rheumatic aches, pains, stiffness and inflammation in muscles and joints. It is still being used today. Hyssop tea can be taken one to three times a day for rheumatic bouts.

Uses Through the Ages. Hyssop has been used to treat discomfort from uterine fibroids. It is also recommended for inflamed mucous conditions throughout the body. Hippocrates recommended it as a remedy for pleurisy. It's antiviral, to fight herpes simplex.

Beneficent Parts: Leaves, Flowers, Stems

Properties: Volatile Oil, Flavonoids, Tannins, Bitter

Values: Expectorant, Pectoral, Stimulant, Carminative, Antiviral, Diaphoretic, Vermifuge

❧

JUNIPER BERRIES   *Juniperus communis*
The Purifying Fruit

This bushy shrub is a member of the pine family and a native of Europe, North Africa, northern Asia, and North America. It has slim, prickly needles on short, spiky stems, and blooms with small pink-to-purple flowers. Round berries grow along the stems, and take two or three years to ripen from green to blue, when they are harvested.

Acid Wastes. Juniper berries filter acid wastes from the body, which is very helpful for excessive acid conditions such as arthritis, rheumatism, and gout. You can get the benefits by doing it the Egyptian way, as a bath.

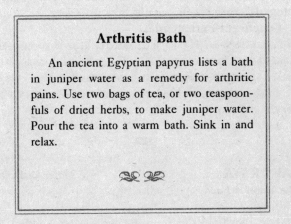

Arthritis Bath

An ancient Egyptian papyrus lists a bath in juniper water as a remedy for arthritic pains. Use two bags of tea, or two teaspoonfuls of dried herbs, to make juniper water. Pour the tea into a warm bath. Sink in and relax.

Athlete's Foot. Juniper berries are an antifungal treatment for athlete's foot. Use two bags of tea or two teaspoons of dried herb to make juniper water. Soak your feet up to the ankles every day until the problem is resolved.

Herpes Simplex Eruptions. Juniper berries are a disinfectant for herpes eruptions. You can use a poultice of the herb right on the site, or take a sitz bath in a potent dose of juniper tea. The tea can also be used as a skin wash.

Scalp (Dry and Itchy). A rinse with juniper berries tea is a remedy for dry, itchy scalps.

Urinary Tract Infections. A tea of antiseptic juniper berries twice a day is an old-time remedy for urinary tract infections and cystitis. It has also been used to treat painful urination and incontinence.

Yeast Infections. A douche with juniper berries tea brings top-notch relief for vaginitis and yeast.

Caution: This herb can cause kidney irritation with prolonged internal use. The best use is short term, or external. Avoid if you have kidney disorders.

Beneficent Part: Berries

Properties: Vitamins A, B3, B-Complex, C, E, K, Magnesium, Iron, Sulfur, Phosphorus, Selenium, Sodium, Zinc, Calcium, Potassium, Manganese—Volatile Oil, Flavonoids, Glycosides, Tannins

Values: Antiseptic, Digestive Tonic, Antirheumatic, Antitumor, Diuretic, Carminative

⁌⁍

KAVA KAVA   *Piper methysticum*
The Mood Adjuster

This root from the South Pacific was once called "an intoxicating pepper" by explorer Captain Cook because it made his sailors seem like they were drunk. It's a tall, leafy shrub and member of the pepper family with a history of use in ceremonies in the South Pacific for heightening the senses of hearing and sight. Kava kava is a mild sedative that creates a tranquil feeling that reputedly does not lead to any loss in concentration or change in motor reflexes. Kavalcones in the root are credited with its calming effect. It can ease heart palpitations; relax the muscles; relieve anxiety, tension, and emotional stress. In the South Pacific, the islanders chewed the root, and saliva is needed to break down kava kava for the best results.

Caution: High doses can be intoxicating.
Beneficent Part: Root

❧

LAVENDER
The Herb of Harmony

Lavandula officinale

At home in woody terrain in the western Mediterranean, lavender is cultivated in Europe, Africa, and the United States. There are twenty-eight species with variations in the leaves, and flowers that range in color from an Alpine white to purple-blue, but none can capture the aromatic and medicinal value of the official lavender. It's a shrubby plant with short, irregular stems; slim, straight leaves; and long-stemmed spikes that bloom at the top with whorls of tiny purple aromatic flowers. It has remained one of the most treasured herbs from ancient to modern times.

Medicinal Perfume

The French cultivate lavender to use its essential oil for perfumes, and the women who wear lavender may not realize why they feel calmer, are less likely to faint or experience headaches. Lavender is a tonic for the nerves and remedy for tension headaches.

When women use lavender sachet in their clothing drawers, they are getting more than perfume. Lavender is antiseptic and antibacterial.

In Spain and Portugal, lavender flowers were scattered on the floors of homes and churches for celebrations. Was it only for the scent? Lavender lifts the spirits, fights viruses including pneumonia, and keeps flies and mosquitoes away.

In old England, lavender was used in bonfires to banish *evil spirits*—that meant viruses, bacteria, and the plague. In France it was used to fight cholera.

Lavender is one of three herbs that the Pilgrims carried to America to guard their health in the new world.

Anxiety, Tension, Headaches, Nerves on Edge. Calming lavender tea is particularly attuned to the brain to relieve stress, headaches, anxiety, depression, mood swings, dizziness, and fainting. It steadies your nerves and invigorates you. The first Queen Elizabeth of England took lavender tea for headaches.

Facial Steam Treatment. One of the best skin healers, antiseptic lavender disinfects acne blemishes and stimulates repair of tissues. A tea bag of lavender, or the dried herbs in boiling water, can be used for a lavender facial steam treatment to cleanse and comfort problem skin.

Infectious Diseases and Fevers. Lavender tea reduces fevers, detoxifies your body, and induces sweating to eliminate the toxins. It's a potent antiseptic and was used to fight diphtheria, typhoid, streptococcus, and pneumonia. It's a good tea to keep on hand to take for those sudden fevers of unknown origin. It could keep you on your feet while you get to the hospital.

Lice. Lavender tea can be used as a scalp wash to kill lice. You can dot it on hot spots on your pet, for lice. It gives them a dreamy scent.

Mouth and Throat. Lavender tea used as a gargle is a remedy for toothaches, sore throats, and laryngitis. It provides antiseptic protection to fight infections.

Purify the Air. Beat midwinter blues and purify musty, unhealthy air with a tea bag of lavender in water

Nirvana Bath

Lavender, from the Latin *lavare*, means "to wash"—and that means body, mind, and spirit. Lavender caresses your skin while it disinfects, it calms your nerves, settles your digestion, brings harmony while you soak. It soothes bruises, reduces puffiness, and leaves your skin scented like a piney breeze. The Romans used it in their baths to feel rejuvenated.

To experience the nirvana, use two tea bags of lavender in a pot of boiling water, let them steep for a minute, then add the water and tea bags to a hot bath. It costs a mere fraction of lavender bath salts or lavender bath sachets, but more important, the natural herb teas have no chemicals, additives, or dyes. You get all of the medicinal benefits of pure lavender to penetrate your skin. A great bath to use for recovery from an illness, surgery, or chronic exhaustion.

at a slow boil on your stove. Its powerful antiseptic cleanses the air and its aromatic scent lifts your spirits.

Vomiting and Diarrhea. Lavender tea can ease vomiting and diarrhea while you call the doctor. A good tea to pack for travel, for emergency treatment.

Wounds. Lavender tea is an antiseptic water that can be used as a healing wash for wounds.

Beneficent Part: Flowers

Properties: Volatile Oil, Tannins, Coumarins, Flavonoids, Triterpenoids

Values: Analgesic, Antibacterial, Antiseptic, Antispasmodic, Carminative, Relaxant, Nerve Tonic

❧

LEMON   *Citrus limon*
The Fantastic Fruit

The lemon's origins are not certain, but it is pre-
sumed to be a native of India and Europe. Its virtues are
simply fabulous. High in vitamin C and bioflavonoids to
fight infections; prevent thickening of arterial walls;
strengthen veins, blood vessels, capillaries; prevent
bruising and varicose veins. It has vitamins A, B1, B2, B3,
and mucilage. It's antiseptic, antirheumatic, antibacterial,
antioxidant; reduces fevers and removes acid wastes from
the body. The lemon may seem acidic, but its nature in
your system is alkaline. Lemon is an ideal flavoring for a
tea, but it can also be a tea on its own. In France and
England, lemon in hot water with sugar is a time-honored treatment for coughs and colds.

Beneficent Parts: Fruit, rind, juice, oil

❧

LEMON BALM   *Melissa officinalis*
The Nerve Balm

This native of southern Europe has mint-green heart-
shaped leaves with crinkled tops and serrated edges. It
blooms in late summer with small white flowers. *Melissa*
in Greek means "honey bee," and lemon balm has many
of the tonic qualities as the queen bee's favorite royal

jelly. Once called *Cure-All*, lemon balm was popular in potions to preserve youthfulness. If you break a leaf, you will be treated to a lemon scent that lifts your spirits.

Special Feature: Nature's Antihistamine

Allergies and Asthma. Iced lemon balm tea relieves tension and aids respiratory healing. It's a wholesome tea you can take regularly for antiviral and antibacterial protection to keep allergic "attacks" at bay. When you get a cold or flu, hot lemon balm tea will help you sweat out the toxins.

Beeee Happy. Lemon balm is an antidepressant and tonic for your nervous system. Take it as an iced tea to alleviate tension and anxiety if you struggle with nervous disorders or nervous exhaustion. It's particularly attuned to your kidneys and urinary tract to cleanse toxins and renew strength. It will get you buzzing around again with more vitality.

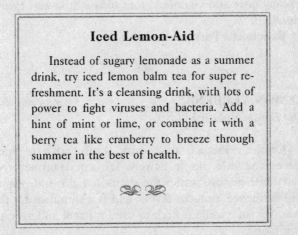

Iced Lemon-Aid

Instead of sugary lemonade as a summer drink, try iced lemon balm tea for super refreshment. It's a cleansing drink, with lots of power to fight viruses and bacteria. Add a hint of mint or lime, or combine it with a berry tea like cranberry to breeze through summer in the best of health.

Digestive Distress. Lemon balm soothes the entire digestive tract to relieve spasms, indigestion, gas, and colic. It's a happy herb to take for stress-related disorders, including colitis, since it helps you to feel calmer all over, and that's a healthy feeling.

Beneficent Part: Leaves

Properties: Volatile Oil, Polyphenols (Fights Strep), Tannins, Bitter Principle, Flavonoids, Rosmarinic Acid, Triterpenoids, Analgesic

Values: Antidepressant, Antihistamine, Antibacterial, Antiviral, Eases Spasms, Nervous System Tonic, Aromatic, Digestive Stimulant, Eases Tension in Peripheral Blood Vessels

❧

LEMONGRASS
An Enhancer for Blends

Lemongrass is an aromatic herb that you'll often find in blends. It is used to harmonize the flavor, since it has a lemony taste and vitamin C that adds a little zest to any blend.

Beneficent Part: Leaves

❧

LEMON VERBENA   *Lippia citriodora*
The Lemon Sedative

Lemon verbena is an aromatic shrub with pale green leaves and pale purple flowers. It's a fragrant sedative that eases spasms, settles the stomach, fights indigestion and flatulence, reduces fevers, and is a stimulant for the skin. It's an excellent herb to use for flavor and synergy in a blend.

Beneficent Parts: Leaves and flowers

❧

LICORICE
Glycyrrhiza glabra
The Soother

This woody perennial can be six feet tall in its home in the wilds of southeast Europe and southwest Asia, but it is now cultivated in many warm climates. It has a bright green stem, dark green oval leaves, with flowers shaped like peas, in mauve or cream colors. It has a big tap root, with long branch roots or "runners" that can spread to three feet.

Adrenal Stimulant. Licorice is a tonic for the adrenal glands, which produce the "fight-or-flight" hormones for coping with stress. Weak adrenals are associated with constant fatigue, bouts of depression and irritability, muscle weakness, indigestion, inadequate nutrient assimilation, and lack of concentration. One way to help your adrenal glands get the boost they need is a cup of licorice tea.

Allergies, Asthma, Hay Fever. Licorice contains glycyrrhizin which has antiallergic value similar to cortisone, but without side effects. A cup of licorice tea can ease allergic symptoms and soothe the respiratory tract to reduce inflammation. It's a mild expectorant to clear phlegm. The ancient Greeks used licorice to treat asthma.

Indigestion. Licorice is a sweet, soothing tea to take for indigestion.

Stomach Ulcers. Licorice helps to reduce the acid secretions in the stomach and provides a protective mucous for the stomach lining. It is a well-known remedy for ulcers.

Uses Through the Ages. Licorice has been used medicinally for thousands of years to tone the spleen, to benefit Chi, to stop coughs, soothe the lungs, clear heat from the body, and as a detoxifier.

Special Feature: A Natural Steroid

Research on glycyrrhizin shows that it is broken down in digestion to produce an anti-inflammatory action like cortisone without side effects. It's antiallergic and antiarthritic. Licorice tea can be used for inflammatory pain, arthritis, and allergies.

Caution: Avoid licorice if you have hypertension, heart problems, thyroid problems, or kidney disorders. Glycyrrhizin in licorice can cause heartburn, edema, headaches, and cardiac problems in high doses. You can find licorice without glycyrrhizin in the European varieties, where it is removed from the root for medicinal use.

Beneficent Part: Root

Properties: Vitamins A, B-Complex, B2, B3, B5, C (Flavonoids), E; Good Source of Iron, Magnesium, Potassium, Silicon, Sodium; Also Calcium, Lecithin, Selenium, Zinc, Glycyrrhizin Triterpenoid Saponins, Bitter Principle, Asparagin, Coumarins, Tannins, Volatile Oil, Estrogenic Isoflavones

Values: Anti-inflammatory, Antipyretic, Expectorant, Diuretic

LINDEN BLOSSOMS   *Tilia europaea*
A Bouquet for Blends

Linden blossoms are tenderhearted flowers with a delicate bouquet and calming nature. They make a soothing tea to reduce internal stress, relieve anxiety, and reduce muscle tension. The flowers have a calming effect on your heart to ease palpitations. You'll often find linden blossoms in blends for their harmonizing effect on other herbs and their unique flavor.

Beneficent Part: Flowers

LUNGWORT
Pulmonaria officinalis
The Herb for the Lungs

This Mediterranean member of the borage family prefers woods and shade and is distinguished by its decorative leaves which are rough, oval, and speckled with white. Its buds are red, but the flowers open in pale purple.

In herbal tradition, a plant's value to the human body was literally "read" in its appearance, and it was believed that the white speckles on lungwort's leaves mirrored the appearance of the lungs. This gave the herb its Latin name, *pulmonaria*, or lung plant.

Lung Weakness. Lungwort is one of the most esteemed herbs for cleansing the lungs and respiratory tract. The mucous lining of your lungs acts as a barrier to prevent infections and diseases from penetrating into the lung tissue. Lungwort has a soothing mucilage that coats and protects the mucous lining of the lungs, which can ease many disorders associated with weakness in the lungs, including allergies, asthma, bronchitis, shortness of breath, wheezing, lingering respiratory infections, repetitive coughs and colds. Semiannual cleansing with lungwort tea is a health treatment for your pulmonary system.

Beneficent Part: Leaves

Properties: Keratin, Vitamin C, B-Complex, Iron, Copper, Silver, Manganese, Titanium, Nickel

Values: Emollient, Pectora, Expectorant, Mucilaginous, Tonic, Mild Astringent, Demulcent

❧

MA HUANG (see EPHEDRA)
MARIGOLD (see CALENDULA)

Pulmonary Cleansing Tea

Vigorous—One cup of lungwort tea two or three times a day for a week to cleanse, decongest, and soothe the mucous membranes of your lungs. *Moderate*—One cup of lungwort tea once a day for two or three weeks.

MARSHMALLOW   *Althea officinalis*
The Herb of Plenty

Indigenous to the fields, marshes, salt meadows and riverbanks of China and Europe, marshmallow is one of one thousand species of mallows. It has thick stems, rough leaves, and it blooms with big pink-to-red flowers. Its name *Althea* is derived from the Greek *altho*, which means "to cure."

Here's a little rhyme to help you remember the uses of marshmallow, which are plentiful:

> *Dry places are moistened*
> *Hard conditions are softened*
> *Inflammation goes away*
> *Tissues resist decay*

Special Feature: Excellent Anti-inflammatory Inside and Out

1. Inflammatory Conditions. Take marshmallow tea internally for any inflammatory condition to speed relief. It's a wholesome brew that carries a lot of healing power.

2. Poultice for Inflammation. Arab physicians used marshmallow leaves as a poultice for inflammations. You can make an instant herb poultice by adding a small amount of warm water to the dried herb or by breaking open a tea bag for the herb. Let the herb steep like a tea for a few minutes. You will feel the soothing mucilage when you pick up the warm herb in your fingers. Apply it to any site of an inflammation, cover it with a clean bandage, and let it do its job.

Immunity, Antiaging, and Disease Resistance. Marshmallow is an oxygenator that helps to fight cellular aging and decay. It has been called *Mortification Root*, for its ability to prevent tissue decay. Internally and externally, hardened areas are softened, dry areas are moistened, and inflammation is relieved. It contains a healing mucilage that coats and protects the mucous membranes of your body from your respiratory tract to your intestines, where it soothes and protects the intestinal lining to fight intestinal disorders and colitis. It has strong nutritional value, with iron for the blood, calcium for the bones, keratin for the hair, silica for tissue repair, and *asparagine*, which strengthens the kidneys, fights cystitis, painful urination, and bladder irritations. It's a wonderful tea to take routinely for health and disease prevention. It can help to keep you fit as you age. In France, the flowers are used in a tea—*tisane de quatre fleurs*—for a cold remedy.

Kidney Weakness. Kidney irritations can be treated naturally with a cup of marshmallow tea two times a day for five days. Break for a few days, then continue with the treatment.

Muscles, Sinews (Aches and Pains). Marshmallow

Mellow Mallow Tea

Marshmallow tea is a generous brew with lots of nutrients to strengthen your immunity and improve your overall health. Many old herbals say: A spoonful of marshmallow a day keeps disease away. The taste is plain, but you can charm it with a spritz of orange.

꧁꧂

---

tea is especially good for aches and pains in muscles and sinews. It eases inflammation and speeds healing of the area.

Non-Insulin-Dependent Diabetes. Marshmallow helps to lower blood sugar levels, and has been used as a tea for non-insulin-dependent diabetes.

Protein for Vegetarians and Muscle Builders. Marshmallow has easy-to-assimilate proteins, which makes it a valuable tea, hot or iced, for vegetarians and muscle builders.

Throat Inflammation, Larynx, Laryngitis, Bronchitis. Take marshmallow tea for laryngitis, bronchitis, and larynx and throat inflammations. Its soothing mucilage coats the area to reduce inflammation and speed healing.

Wounds and Benign Growths. Marshmallow can be used as an external poultice on hardened areas such as old wounds and benign growths to help to prevent mortification or decay of tissues. It softens and moistens hardened areas and helps to restore healthy tissue. If the area has an infection, combine with slippery elm to draw out toxins.

Uses Through the Ages. Marshmallow leaves were eaten as a vegetable in ancient Rome, and considered a delicacy. They are still used today for spring salads in France. In China, it is a food herb—the root is boiled first, then fried with onions and butter.

Beneficent Parts: Root, leaves, flowers

Properties: High in Vitamins A, B1, B2, B3, B5, C, Asparagine, Oxygen, Calcium, Cellulose, Iodine, Iron, Keratin, Magnesium, Manganese, Mucilage, Pectin, Phosphorus, Potassium, Silicon, Starch, Sodium, Sugar

Values: Very Emollient, Very Demulcent, Mucilaginous, Diuretic

❧

MEADOWSWEET   *Spiraea ulmaria*
The Acid Reliever

This European native has dark green leaves with fancy serrated edges and a scent like almond. It blooms with close clusters of small, cream-colored flowers. Called *Queen of the Meadow*, *Bridewort*, and *Lady of the Meadow*, it was a sacred herb of the Druids.

Acid Reflux and Digestive Distress. Meadowsweet is a tasty, gentle tea that relieves stomach acidity and calms your digestive tract. It has a soothing mucilage that coats and protects the lining of your digestive tract. It's an *alternative* herb—one that will subtly and gently restore health to your digestive tract over time.

Eyes (Burning and Itching). A tea from meadowsweet flowers makes an excellent eyewash to take the sting and itch from irritated eyes.

Special Feature: Nature's "Aspirin"

Meadowsweet is the herb that first brought "salicylates" to the world's attention, when they were extracted

Recuperation Tea

Meadowsweet tea with honey is a gentle remedy to restore health and vitality after an illness. It was revered in old England, and was even mentioned by Chaucer as one of fifty herbs that was used in a drink called *Save*.

in the 1830s. In the 1890s, Bayer created the synthetic version of salicylates with acetylsalicylates—or aspirin. While aspirin can cause gastric bleeding and gastric distress if it is taken routinely, the natural salicylates in meadowsweet are not known to produce these side effects, since the herb's other properties cool and harmonize the salicylates' action in your system. In fact, the herb meadowsweet is actually a remedy for gastric disorders!

Caution: Avoid meadowsweet if you can't take salicylates or aspirin.

Beneficent Parts: Leaves and flowers

Properties: Volatile Oil, Citric Acid, Flavonoids, Salicylates, Mucilage, Tannins

Values: Digestive Remedy, Aromatic, Astringent, Anti-inflammatory, Antirheumatic, Diuretic, Fever Reducer

MILK THISTLE
Also called SILYMARIN
The Herb of Renewal

Silybum marianum

This ten-foot-tall member of the daisy family is at home among hedges and in wastelands of western and central Europe and Mediterranean regions. It has deep green glossy leaves with milk-white veins and prickly tips. It blooms from long stems with cone-shaped flowers that are purple-red.

Once called *Our Lady's Thistle*, it was believed that milk from the Virgin Mary fell on the thistle's leaves to give them their milk-white veins.

Liver Strength and Renewal. This is a valuable herb to strengthen your liver, which in turn can boost your resistance to disease and help you recover from illnesses more quickly. Your liver plays an important role in immunity. It manufactures chemicals to clean your blood. It helps to detoxify your system of harmful chemicals, pollutants, and metabolic wastes. It secretes bile which stimulates digestive juices that help to break down nutrients from foods into an absorbable form that can be used by your cells. It helps to regulate proteins, recycle hormones, and dissolve fat-soluble toxins. When your liver is sluggish or "stagnated," the health of your whole system is compromised. Many everyday problems are linked to liver deficiency, including recurring headaches, skin problems, depression, poor circulation, chronic fatigue, indigestion, irritability, mood swings, lack of concentration, and diminished resistance to disease. More advanced liver disorders can result from excessive use of alcohol, drugs, and medications that have liver damage as side effects.

Milk thistle contains *silymarin*, a unique combination of flavonolignans that protect liver cells from damage by free radicals and toxins. In German studies, when potent

liver poisons were tested against silymarin, it was found
that silymarin prevented the poisons from entering liver
cells, and it fragmented other poisons before they could
cause damage. It is the only known natural compound
that protects liver cells and renews liver vitality, even
during disease states.

Annual Treatment for Liver and Spleen. A thirty-
day treatment with milk thistle tea can help to rid your
system of toxins, tone your liver, and improve your vital
energy and immunity. It's a gentle, wholesome drink
that you can take to boost your strength during an illness,
or to recover from long periods of exhaustion or chronic
fatigue. It's a great tea for golden-age people to revitalize
their liver energy.

Depression. If you suffer from depression, try milk
thistle as a routine tea for liver energy. One of the or-
ganic causes of depression is liver deficiency. Melancholy, once thought of as a "woman's complaint," is
often a condition of the liver that can be improved with
milk thistle tea. One herbal says that milk thistle "makes
a man merry as a cricket."

Headaches. If you are prone to recurring headaches,
milk thistle tea could be the boost you need to keep
headaches away, since liver weakness is linked to headaches.

"Recovery" Treatments. Milk thistle tea can be a
vital aid in recovery programs, including:

1. Withdrawal from alcohol or drugs
2. To recover from the side effects of liver-damaging
   medications
3. To recover from chemotherapy or radiation treatments—milk thistle is used in China as an adjunct to
   chemotherapy to insure minimal damage to the liver
   for patients
4. To aid recovery from liver diseases

Skin Abscesses, Eruptions. Milk thistle tea makes

an effective skin wash to cleanse toxins from problem sites. Also take the tea internally to help to resolve these disorders from the inside.

Toxic Poisoning. An old Saxon saying claims that milk thistle will set snakes to flight. Since snakes are carriers of venom or poisons, the Saxon saying was right on target. Milk thistle tea will help to protect your liver cells against damage, in the event of toxic poisoning or toxic exposure.

Special Feature: Antiallergenic

Milk thistle helps to suppress the release of histamines in your body, which are linked to allergic reactions and headaches.

Beneficent Parts: Whole herb—roots, leaves, seeds, hulls

Properties: Silymarin Antioxidants, Silybine

Values: Liver Strength, Antiallergenic, Antitoxin, Antiaging

&

MINT (see PEPPERMINT)

&

MOTHERWORT   *Leonurus cardiaca*
The Herb That Comforts the Heart

This European native is a time-honored herb with a very decisive stature. A strong, thick stem shoots straight up, large three-lobed leaves shoot straight out, in opposites on the stem. At the bases of the leaves, delicate hooded flowers bloom around the stem—pale pink outside and purple inside.

Menopause, Menses. Motherwort's nature for soothing and calming the nervous system, maintaining the health of the heart, and its beneficial effects on women's

reproductive systems makes it a "mothering" tea for
menses problems and menopause. You might want to
sweeten it with honey, since the taste is superbly bitter.

Nervous Disorders. A cup of motherwort tea quiets
the nervous system and can be used to ease the aches of
neuralgia and all nervous conditions.

Palpitations of the Heart. Motherwort's name
cardiaca comes from its value as a heart tonic. It contains
calcium chloride which calms the heart and eases palpitations.

Spinal Disorders. Motherwort tea is a tonic for the
spine and nerves, and can be used to ease discomfort
from spinal disorders.

Tremors. Motherwort tea stops internal tremors by
soothing the entire nervous system.

Uses Through the Ages. In China, Motherwort is
called *Tsan Ts'ai* and is used for menstrual disorders, to
tone the liver and improve vision.

Beneficent Parts: Flowers, leaves, stems

Properties: Volatile Oil, Vitamin A, Alkaloids, Bitter Glycosides,
Tannins

Values: Cardiac Tonic, Antispasmodic, Nervine, Diaphoretic, Uterine Stimulant, Sedative, Emmenagogue, Carminative

❧

MULLEIN   *Verbascum thapus*
A Respiratory Sweetheart

Once called *Lady's Foxglove*, mullein is a big plant
that has large, oblong leaves with a pebble finish and
woolly hairs. It blooms from long spikes with densely
packed, bright yellow flowers. Mullein is a sweet-
natured, calming herb that charms any health blend. It's
a gentle expectorant with a sedative nature and soothing
mucilage for the lungs and respiratory tract. It is a

marvelous tea to use for respiratory weakness, including chronic coughs, congestion, colds, lung weakness, breathing difficulties, asthma, and bronchitis. Mullein is a good source of vitamins including flavonoids, it has saponins for cleansing the body, and its flowers are antibacterial. It's food for the glands, including the testicles and ovaries, and it has anti-inflammatory properties to reduce glandular swellings.

Special Feature: Mullein tea is a great rinse to brighten blond hair.

Beneficent Parts: Leaves and flowers

꿏

NETTLE (STINGING)   *Urtica dioica*
The Sting That Brings Energy

Flourishing everywhere, nettle has heart-shaped leaves with serrated edges, small greenish flowers, and a fruit with one seed. The male and female flowers are separated on the plant. Above all things, nettle is known for its sting. When you touch a leaf, histamines and fornic acids can give you a stinging feeling. A story about nettle's sting illustrates how legends and folklore reveal the secrets of plants to new generations.

Legend tells that Roman nettle was planted in England by Caesar's soldiers, whose flimsy uniforms weren't warm enough for the raw climate of England. When their legs went numb from cold, the soldiers whipped their legs with nettle to sting them to life. If this were simply a story about soldiers whipping themselves into action whatever way they could, any plant would do, but they used nettle. Was there something special about nettle's properties that penetrated the soldiers' skins?

Blood Tonic and Circulatory Stimulant. Nettle is a

blood tonic that stimulates circulation, gets the blood going to extremities, and gets you on your feet again. It's a good tea to take to recover from an injury that limits your mobility, for the elderly to improve circulation, and for aches in the limbs and joints from arthritis, rheumatism, gout.

Energy Builder. Nettle is an excellent source of chlorophyll, and it carries a healthy reserve of vitamins and minerals, including vitamins A, C, D, and K; choline; lecithin; silica; iron (a red blood builder). It's beneficial to the liver, gallbladder, and kidneys. It's a tea to build your energy.

Respiratory Weakness. Nettle is antiseptic to fight infections. It's a good tea for respiratory weakness, shortness of breath, coughs, colds, and congestion. It has been used to treat asthma, allergies, and hay fever, but since nettle contains histamines, it would be best to have professional guidance if you want to try nettle for allergic conditions.

Special Feature: Nettle has serotonin, for healthy brain function, to help to regulate moods.

Beneficent Parts: Root, leaves, and stem

Properties: Vitamins, Minerals, Acetylcholine, Histamine, Fornic Acid, Glucoquinones, Serotonin, Tannins

Values: Astringent, Blood Tonic, Circulatory Stimulant, Diuretic, Lowers Blood Sugar

❧

OATSTRAW   *Avena sativa*
The Body Tonic

A native of Europe and the United States, the slender stalks with drooping husks are a familiar power food—oatmeal cereal is made from the crushed grain, oat bran is made from the husks, and has been credited with lowering cholesterol levels. The medicinal version—oat-straw—uses the whole plant, dried and chopped to make a total health tea.

Body Tonic for Vital Energy. Oatstraw tea is a full-body tonic to strengthen your immunity and build your energy. It can help to stabilize your thyroid function, regulate blood sugar, reduce cholesterol levels, and bathe your nervous system in nutrients for health and harmony. It's a sweet, wholesome tea with lots of antioxidant power, antibiotic properties, and it's an antidepressant. Use it as a routine tea to fight exhaustion and fatigue, for recovery from illness, to resist stress, combat anxiety, depression, insomnia, and for natural resistance to disease.

Multiple Sclerosis. Oatstraw tea has been used to help fight the debilitating effects of multiple sclerosis. It is also excellent for arthritis, rheumatism and bursitis.

Skin. Oatstraw tea has vitamins A, D, and E; zinc; and silicon which makes it a power tea for your skin. The tea can also be used as a healing wash for problem areas on your skin, since oatstraw has natural antibiotic properties.

Beneficent Part: Whole plant

Properties: Vitamins A, D, B1, B2, E, Calcium, Iron, Selenium, Silicon, Magnesium, Manganese, Zinc—Alkaloids, Saponins, Steroidal Compounds, Carotene, Wheat Protein, Starch, Fat

Values: Stimulant, Nerve Tonic, Antibiotic, Antioxidant, Antispasmodic, Diuretic, Diaphoretic, Carminative

❧

OOLONG (see GREEN)

❧

ORANGE, BITTER
The Tonic Fruit

Citrus aurantium
Citrus reticulata

Bitter orange is a native of China, where it is considered to be a "Chi" tonic that moves stagnant energy and eases digestive distress, including indigestion, constipation, and bloating. It contains vitamins A, B, C, and flavonoids and has expectorant properties to remove phlegm. It soothes the nervous system and it's a *carminative herb*—one that eases spasms. It's reputed to be helpful to dissolve kidney stones.

Beneficent Parts: Fresh fruit, dried fruit, peel

෨෩

PAPAYA
Also called PAW PAW
The Digestive Regulator

Carica papaya

This tree from the West Indies and South America resembles a palm, has seven-lobed leaves, and produces an oblong, yellow-orange, melonlike fruit. It has also been called *Melon Tree*.

Digestive Health. Papaya is a top-notch tea for digestive disorders. It contains enzymes for healthy digestion and assimilation of nutrients, including the powerful papain to digest proteins, pepsin to digest vegetables, an enzyme to digest milk proteins, and one for starches. It also counters acidity which eases gastrointestinal distress, acid reflux, indigestion, and constipation. Papaya is a 16th century remedy for gastrointestinal distress, and it's still one of the best!

Heart. Papaya contains an alkaloid carpain which is good for the health of the heart.

Lymph System. Papaya cleanses the lymph system and fights infections.

Weight Loss. Weight problems are often related to digestive difficulties, gastrointestinal distress, constipation, and waste stagnation. A good first step to weight regulation is to get your gastrointestinal system in fit shape. Everything works better when the processes of digestion, assimilation, and elimination of wastes are more stabilized.

Beneficent Parts: Fruit, leaves, seeds, juice

Properties and Values Listed Above

✻

PARSLEY   *Apium petroselinum*
The Green Goddess   *Apium sativum*

Parsley is a winner when it comes to wholesome brews and healing virtues. It's a superior cleanser for the glands, liver, and gallbladder. It's a tonic for the skin, arteries, and capillaries, and has mild antibiotic properties to fight infections. It carries a hearty share of disease-fighting nutrition, including plenty of vitamins A and C antioxidants, protein, B-complex, chlorophyll for the cells, selenium for your natural disease barrier, silicon for tissue repair, and zinc. At the first sign of an illness, parsley tea will give you a jump-start to recovery.

Parsley is also a natural antihistamine. It's an ideal tea for people with asthma, allergies, hay fever, and headaches. Grow your own, or buy it fresh, and use the greens in your tea infuser for a burst of parsley pleasure. In the summer, iced parsley tea will cool you all over and keep allergic reactions at bay. It's a marvelous tea to take routinely to keep you feeling invigorated.

Beneficent Parts: Root, leaves, and seeds

✻

PASSION FLOWER   *Passiflora incarnata*
The Herb of Tranquillity

Passion flower is a beautiful twining vine from the West Indies, also called *May Pop* or *Ancient Vine*. It has three-fingered light green leaves and slim tendrils that seek out something to wrap around and cling to. Its life force is so vital, if you unwrap a tendril, you can literally watch it move in search of something else to cling to. It flowers with exotic purple blossoms that have a fringed center.

Passion flower has an equally passionate symbolism. The Jesuits called it *flower of the five passions* and believed that it was the flower that grew on the cross, in St. Francis of Assisi's vision of Calvary. The five sepals and five petals represented ten apostles, the flower's fringed crown was the crown of thorns, and the five stamens were the five wounds.

Nerve Conditioner. Passion flower improves circulation to your nerves and tones your sympathetic nervous system. It's mildly sedative to relieve pain, antispasmodic to relieve muscle spasms, and a mild relaxant. Passion flower tea can be used for all nervous disorders, including: nervous tension, hyperactivity, irritability, twitching, anxiety, agitation, stress-induced disorders, tension headaches, nervous coughs, exhaustion. It has no side effects. You can take passion flower tea for insomnia, and won't feel drowsy when you wake. Use it as a routine tea, and gradually you'll find that your nerves are steadier, you respond better to stress, and your sleep comes more naturally. It's mildly euphoric.

Uses Through the Ages. It has been used as a treatment for alcoholism. Its Harmala chemical is known to dilate coronary arteries for heart health.

Special Features: Kills mold, fungus, and is antibacterial

Beneficent Parts: Vine and flowers

Properties: Harmala Alkaloids, Sugar, Gum, Sterols, Flavonoids, Vitamins A and C, High Calcium, Magnesium

Values: Pain Reliever, Sedative, Relaxant, Nervine, Diuretic, Antispasmodic, Mild Euphoric

☙

PAU D'ARCO
Tabebuia impetiginosa
The Divine Bark

A native to rain forests in Central and South America, the pau d'arco tree has vivid green, oval-shaped leaves with thick golden seams that cut mosaic designs into each serrated leaf. The tree blooms with clusters of dangling purple trumpet flowers.

Early medicine men peeled the tree's bark in long strips. They separated the outer bark from the purple inner bark to make a tea from the inner bark that was a panacea for many maladies for centuries.

Called *The Divine Tree* by the Incas, the bark tea from pau d'arco has been touted as a cure-all in Brazil, Argentina, Mexico, and the Bahamas. While many plants are credited with radiance or a special light which gives them their "divine" status, pau d'arco is said to attract alpha rays that exert a positive electrical charge on human cells. It has crystalline oxygen locked in its inner bark. Pau d'arco is called *Lapacho Morado* by the Spanish, *Taheebo* or "purple bow stick" by the Indians, and in Peru, it is called *Palo de Arco*, which means "to have strength and vigor."

Bark With a Bite. Pau d'arco is packed with nutrients, including iron; calcium; selenium; vitamins A, B-complex, and C; magnesium; manganese; zinc; phosphorous; potassium; and sodium. But that's not all. Its special properties are quite inclusive. It's antibiotic, antibacterial, antiviral, antimicrobial, antifungal, and antitumor. This combination gave pau d'arco its reputation as an immune system stimulant and disease fighter.

Blood Conditioner. Pau d'arco has iron to build red blood. It has been shown to improve hemoglobin production and red blood cell corpuscles.

Candida Control. Candida fungi is normally present as bowel flora, but it can get out of control, spread to other areas of the body, and flourish, creating a host of problems that include: indigestion, bloating after eating, gas, constant fatigue, depression, tension, prostate infections, vaginitis, skin infections, throat inflammations, and fungal-based allergies. Candida can run rampant as a result of several factors:

- Repeated use of antibiotics, especially tetracycline. Studies show fungal growth forty-eight hours after taking tetracycline.
- Habitual steroid use, or corticosteroids which suppress immunity.
- Long-term use of birth control pills or estrogen replacement therapy.
- Parasitic infections which compromise immunity.
- Poor diets, especially ones that are high in sweets and alcohol.

Pau d'arco tea fights excess candida growth on four fronts:

1. It's a powerful antifungal and antimicrobial to cleanse your system of fungus and parasitic infections.
2. It's an immune booster that helps your body fight candida.
3. It contains selenium, which is one of your body's natural defenses against rampant candida growth.
4. It has potent nutritional energy to restore your vitality.

Recipe: For candida or yeast, one cup of pau d'arco

tea daily. (Also, you might consider vitamin E for absorption of selenium, acidophilis to restore good intestinal flora, and eat less sugar.) The recommended way to take your cup of tea is in a thermos of water. Sip the beverage in small amounts during the day. That will keep a steady dose of antifungal liquid in your system as your body goes through its daily metabolic process. Drink plenty of water to cleanse your system during the process.

Colon Health. An excellent cleanser, the bark of pau d'arco fights yeast, intestinal infections, and helps to restore colon vitality.

Immunity. In the mid-eighties, test-tube research in Germany showed that pau d'arco stimulated macrophages, granulocytes, and lymphocytes, including T-cells, which help to fortify immunity. Research also identified an antitumor agent, lapachol, which is known to inhibit cancer tumors in mice, and may also inhibit herpes. There are no current studies in the medical establishment proving the same effectiveness in humans. Pau d'arco has been used by AIDS patients to boost immunity and help fight infections that accompany the disease.

Lymph Congestion. A healthy lymph system keeps many diseases at bay. Pau d'arco tea is a lymph and liver cleanser.

Mucous Congestion. Pau d'arco tea clears mucous conditions and fights mucous infections. This is especially valuable during cold and flu season.

Psoriasis, Eczema, Ringworm, Scabies. Pau d'arco tea fights infections and helps to heal skin.

Throat, Mouth, Gums. Pau d'arco tea as a throat and mouth gargle can help to conquer infections in the mouth.

Uses Through the Ages. Pau d'arco has been used in South America to fight a wide range of diseases.

Special Feature: Fungal infections

Pau d'arco's ability to fight fungal and yeast infections is renowned. Excess fungus can create many disorders that often go undiagnosed until they escalate, and many medications can accelerate fungal growth as a side effect or aftereffect. Fungal infections weaken immunity and compromise your health. For its antifungal value alone, pau d'arco is truly the divine tree.

Caution: Seek your doctor's consent if you are considering any complementary herbal therapy for serious diseases such as cancer or AIDS.

Beneficent Part: Inner purple bark

Properties: Flavonoids, Alkaloids, Quinones, Saponins, Vitamins, and Minerals

Values: Antifungal, Antiviral, Antimicrobial, Antitumor, Antibacterial, Immune Stimulant, Nutrition

&

PEPPERMINT   *Mentha piperita*
The Marvel of Menthol

A native of Europe, perennial peppermint likes warm, moist climates, and the rich soil around brooks or streams. It's an aromatic plant that will invigorate you with one cut leaf. It's also called *White Peppermint* or *Mitcham,* from the area in England where it is cultivated for medicine. It has smooth green stems (undertoned red), and lance-shaped green leaves with serrated edges. In July and August, peppermint blooms with dense clusters of tiny violet-colored flowers that form spikes from the upper leaves.

This charming plant produces oil of peppermint, the third most popular oil in the world next to lemon and orange. It's a powerhouse of menthol.

There are more than 210 species of mints, including spearmint, applemint, pineapple mint, red mint, ginger mint, American wild mint, Russian mint, Corsican mint, and many hybrid-garden and wild mints, but the oil from white peppermint is considered the best.

Crowns of Mint

Mint is mentioned in the Bible as one of the herbs that was used for paying taxes. In Greece and Rome, it flavored sauces and wines, and had a special place in festivals. Those crowns on noble heads were often crowns of invigorating mint. The Japanese valued it so highly, they carried peppermint in small, silver boxes that hung from their belts. In the late 1700s, peppermint caught on in Britain, and when it did, the attraction had a lasting impact.

In old England, medicinal plants were grown in gardens in one district, Mitcham in Surrey. To give you an example of how important peppermint became, in 1750 only a few acres in Mitcham were assigned to peppermint. By 1800, 100 acres grew peppermint, and by 1850, the aroma of peppermint covered 500 acres, with mint farms in southern districts as well. Peppermint farms now flourish in France (where it is called Red Mint), the United States, and around the world.

Chest Congestion, Nasal Congestion. A peppermint tea bag in a pot of boiling water on the stove is a menthol inhalant to clear congestion in your nose and chest.

Cure-All. The British take their mint seriously, and often take what is called *The Peppermint Cure*—they drink *peppermint water* or *peppermint spirits* to ward off colds or disease at the onset. You've got it in peppermint tea.

Headaches. Mint is a strong local pain reliever, applied to skin. A warm tea bag on the spot where the headache is most pronounced will bring pain relief. It's also been used in compresses for the pain of rheumatism or neuralgia.

Peppermint Treat

A tall, cool glass of peppermint tea will ease inner tension and boost your energy. It's a great iced tea to take in a thermos in your car for long-distance drives. It relieves stress without putting you to sleep.

❧ ❧

Laryngitis, Bronchitis. A tea bag of peppermint in a pot of boiling water used as an inhalant will ease your throat and clear bronchial tubes.

Nervous Tension/Stress. Peppermint tea calms you all over. It's been used for hysteria and nervous disorders.

Seasickness and Nausea. Take peppermint tea with you when you cruise. The menthol has an anesthetic effect on nerve endings of the stomach, which prevents seasickness and nausea. Drink it iced.

Stomach Cramps. Peppermint tea alleviates sudden pains in the abdomen.

Toothaches and Cavities. Peppermint is a strong antiseptic and anesthetic, which is ideal for the pain of toothaches. Gargle with peppermint tea, and press the wet tea bag right on the aggravated tooth to numb the pain and treat the infection simultaneously.

Uses Through the Ages. Peppermint has been used for palpitations of the heart, cholic, dyspepsia, and flatulence.

Special Feature: Body Odor

For tough or lingering cases of body odor, take peppermint tea internally, and make extra tea to use as an herbal bath.

Beneficent Part: Whole plant flowering

Properties: Volatile Oil of Peppermint, Good Source of Vitamins A and B-Complex, Vitamin C, Carotenoids, Betaine, Choline, Flavonoids, Minerals, Phytol, Tocopherols, Azulenes, Rosmarinic Acid, Tannin

Values: Stimulant, Antispasmodic, Stomachic, Diaphoretic, Antiemetic, Nervine, Antiseptic, Analgesic, Astringent, Decongestant, Tonic, Bitter

❧

PLANTAIN
The Herbal Star

Plantago Major

A well-known roadside and meadow plant, plantain's leaves form a rosette and lie close to the ground. The leaves are oblong, smooth, and thick, with uneven edges. In a British species, called *Buck's Horn*, the leaves lie on the ground in the form of a star. The flower stems are slim spikes that grow right from the root, and bloom along the top with tiny purple-green flowers.

There are more than two hundred species of plantain, many used for medicines, and yet plantain, like dandelion, is often seen as a troublesome weed. A water variety of plantain common to Europe, Asia, and America grows next to forget-me-nots, as if to remind us, *forget me not*.

Plant of Healing

Plantain was one of the nine sacred herbs of the Saxons and was thought to have migrated with the English colonists as they sailed the world. Because it seemed to crop up underfoot wherever the English colonists went, it was often called *Englishman's Foot*, or *White Man's Foot* by the natives.

There's a marvelous American Indian tale about plantain's unique healing power. It goes something like this: A dog one day was stung by a rattlesnake. Juice of plantain and salt were applied to his wound. The dog in agony soon recovered and shook off all traces of his misadventure.

A similar tale from Greece tells of a toad who was bitten by a spider, and shook off all traces of the poison after eating a plantain leaf.

Plantain was a familiar ingredient in early remedies, and many herbalists believed it could cure *all* diseases. In medieval England, it was called *slan-lus*, "plant of healing."

Forget Me Not Tea

Plain plantain tea is one of the finest brews for general health and recovery from illness. The tea has a deep green vegetable taste that is instantly soothing and cooling. It's a decongestant and blood cleaner. It's good for your liver, kidneys, and heart. It's the first tea to remember when you aren't feeling up to par.

✦✦

Blood. Plain plantain tea is one of the best cleansers to remove toxins from the blood.

Colds. For stuffy head colds that come on like a shot and make you feel as if you are "underwater," plantain is the tea to take on the spot to dry out fast. It's an excellent tea for people with allergies or asthma who are allergic to cold medications, and are very congested. It's fast acting! Stay with plantain tea until the congestion is completely cleared, and you'll feel better than you did before the cold.

Deobstruent. Plantain is a *deobstruent*—meaning it unclogs passageways, particularly lung plugs and liver obstructions (imbedded phlegm).

Fungal Infections. Seeds from psyllium plantain contain mucilage which protects mucous linings from fungal infections, including candida albicans. Look for psyllium plantain tea, but if you can't find it, plain plantain leaves as a tea will be very effective.

Hemorrhoids. Take a sitz bath in plantain tea for fast relief. Also take the tea internally to treat the problem inside and out.

Lungs. Plantain is particularly valuable for the lungs, to fight infections and remove phlegm. It's a time-honored remedy for weak lungs, and coughs from lung disorders. It cools and calms the pulmonary system and helps to restore the mucous lining to protect you from future infections.

Mucous Infections and Inflammations. Mucous membrane infections and inflammations can be responsible for a host of health disorders, including:

- Upper respiratory infections that never seem to let up
- Nasal inflammations, sinusitis, ear and throat infections that recur
- Phlegm and phlegm plugs that inhibit breathing
- Spastic colon and mucous colitis conditions that flare up
- Gastroenteritis that influences appetite, digestion, and absorption
- Vaginal infections that recur
- Ulcerous conditions

Plantain is a "specific" for inflamed mucous linings in your body and head. Take it as a tea for infections and congestion from your head to your toes. It depresses mucous secretions, which helps to dry moist, clogged areas where bacteria thrive and create infections. It pulls toxins from tissues and fights infections lingering there. It has silica to repair damaged tissue in mucous linings. It gets your body in better shape to heal itself.

Poison Ivy. A plantain bath stops itching and prevents the spread of poison ivy. It dries and heals.

Prostate Enlargement. Plantain helps to detoxify tissues; dries, cools, cleans passages; and reduces inflammation. It has been used to treat prostate enlargement.

Skin Infections. Plantain stops the spread of skin infections such as scabies, ringworm, shingles (a strain of herpes). Its leaves are known for their ability to detoxify and heal skin wounds, leaving no trace of the misadventure. In old England, skin ointments with plantain were revered, and plain plantain for skin was even mentioned by Shakespeare. Use plantain tea as a skin wash or in a bath for hard-to-heal skin infections.

Spastic Colon (Colitis). Plantain soothes and reduces pain, spasms, inflammation; detoxifies the colon; and promotes healing. Take as a tea.

Venom, Poisons. Plantain works as an antidote to venom and poisons, including spider- and snakebites, by cleaning toxins from your blood. American Indians called it *Snakeweed* and used it successfully as a cure for venomous bites and poisons, including rattlesnake bites. In the event of poisoning, take plantain tea in a strong brew, while you call 911.

Uses Through the Ages. Cool and sympathetic, plantain has been used for infections in the stomach, digestive tract, bowel, urinary tract, and for liver problems. An old herbal claims it will heal most "griefs" that happen to the eyes. The roots have been used to treat kidney disorders.

Beneficent Part: Leaves

Properties: Mucilage, Glycosides, Tannins, Silica, Vitamins C, K, Minerals

Values: Cooling, Detoxifying, Demulcent, Astringent, Wound Healing, Decongestant, Expectorant, Antiseptic, Diuretic

∌

RASPBERRY
The Gravity Reliever

Rubus Idaeus

This native of Europe is a biennial with spreading perennial roots. It's a small shrub that grows very erect, and was once called *Ida*, or *Bramble of Mount Ida*, from Mount Ida in Asia Minor, where it flourished. It flowers in May and June and produces the delectable red raspberry fruit.

Canker Sores, Bleeding Gums. Gargle with raspberry tea for canker sores in the mouth, or bleeding gums. It also helps to remove tartar from teeth.

Diarrhea (Extreme). A good tea to keep on hand for a severe bout of diarrhea that comes on unexpectedly. Take it as an iced tea for diarrhea, and look forward to immediate relief from this rich amber drink.

Nutrition. Raspberry has vitamins A, B-complex, C, E; citric and malic acids; calcium; niacin; iron; magnesium; pectin; potassium; selenium; silicon; sodium; zinc.

Women's Lower Body Stress. Raspberry tones the lower body organs and pelvic muscles, which helps to ease difficulties associated with uterine disorders. It also relieves tension, making it an excellent tea for bearing-down pressure in the lower body. Also strengthens kidneys and urinary tract.

Beneficent parts: Leaves and fruit

Properties: Vitamins and Minerals, Volatile Oils, Tannin, Fruit Acids

Values: Toning, Astringent, Pelvic and Uterine Relaxant, Mucous Cleanser

Vacation Salvation

Cold raspberry tea can save your vacation, in case an intestinal bug gets you! Safe for children to ease stomach complaints. Pack a few tea bags for vacation insurance.

❧❧ ❧❧

❧

RED CLOVER   *Trifolium pratense*
The Herb That Met a Tempest

Common to Europe and Asia, red clover is a plant that pops up in grass or meadows with long stems that rise straight from the root, three-lobed leaves—often seen as three separate leaves—and fragrant oval flowers in hues from red to purple. In medieval England, the three-lobed leaves were linked with the Trinity.

An old herbal notes that the leaves of red clover tremble and stand up against a storm or tempest, and it met a tempest of controversy in the 1940s in the United States, when it was touted as a "wonder herb" that could cure cancer, used in alternative clinics for cancer treatment. While it is still being studied for its toxin-binding properties, the exaggerated claims for red clover as a cancer "cure" caused its reputation to suffer and its real value was clouded over. Prior to that, red clover was used as a tonic for health and respected for its ability to resolve skin disorders.

Red clover is now being used in small amounts in blends, more in keeping with its traditional use.

Coughs, Colds, Bronchitis. Red clover has a long history of use for respiratory infections.

Hair (Dry). Red clover tea can be used as a rinse for dry hair.

Estrogenic. Red clover is reputed to have an estrogenic nature in its flavonoids.

Eye Infections. Red clover tea makes an excellent wash for the eyes, and has been used to fight conjunctivitis.

Skin Infections. Red clover tea is an old-time remedy for persistent skin problems, including eczema and psoriasis. The tea can be used externally as a cleansing wash for the skin.

Beneficent Part: Flowers

Properties: Vitamins A, B-Complex, B2, C; Bioflavonoids; Calcium; Copper; Iron; Magnesium; Manganese; Niacin; Phosphorus; Potassium; Selenium; Silicon; Sodium; Cobalt; Nickel; Tin—Volatile Oil; Phenolic Acids (salicylic); Sitosterols; Starch; Fatty Acids

Values: Alterative, Antiseptic, Anti-inflammatory, Deobstruent, Galactagogue, Nerve Soother, Nutritive, Sedative

◦◦

ROSE HIPS (Wild Dog Rose)   *Rosa canina, rugosa, and centifolia*

From Skin to Spirit, the Perfect Rose
For Young and Old, the Perfect Rose
A Wealth of Health, the Perfect Rose

The home of the rose is thought to be Persia, but the rose is so old, its origins remain a mystery. Thirty-million-year-old fossils of prehistoric roses have been found, predating the dawn of the rose to a million years earlier.

Today, it is estimated that there are more than ten thousand cultivated roses, but the medicinal species are natives of Europe with light green, thorny stems, bright green oval leaves with deep center seams and serrated edges. The blooms can be white, rich pinks, light or sweet reds, with hundreds of petals or only a few petals as in *Rosa rugosa.*

Rose hips are reddish-colored coverings that grow around the real fruits for protection, and for this reason, they are often called "false fruits."

The Queen of the Flowers

According to a Christmas legend, the moment the Christ Child was born, every rose in the world bloomed.

The name *Wild Dog Rose* comes from the rose's earliest use as a remedy for the bites of mad ("wild") dogs.

In ancient Rome, the rose was used as a tribute or blessing. It was strewn in the path of victors, on the floors for feasts, used to decorate warships, worn as garlands, and its petals were floated on wine in winter.

In England, when famine was rampant, rose hips were used for food.

Nutrient Tonic. Rose hips tea has a vital antiaging and invigorating combination of nutrients for immunity and well-being, including: vitamins A and D, B-complex, C—citric, malic, and ascorbic acid, E, K (vitality and longevity), bioflavonoid rutin, calcium, iron, silicon, selenium, naturally occurring sodium for the cells, magnesium, manganese, pectin (fiber), phosphorus, potassium, sulfur, zinc.

Plain and Simple Protection. Rose hips tea is a vibrant drink with lots of healing power. You'll notice how good it makes you feel as you drink it, hot or iced. It's cleansing for your respiratory tract which makes you breathe easier. It's a tonic for energy, so you tire less

---

Perfect Rose, Perfect Tea

Rose hips may be called "false fruits," but not when it comes to their healing virtues. They make a perfect tea to reap the bounty of nature at its finest. The nutrient value of rose hips tea is as rich as the colors of the rose, the brew is deep amber-red, it lifts your spirits as you drink it, and the result is a feeling of well-being!

---

easily. It gives you disease protection, so you aren't as susceptible to every cold and virus. You heal faster. You rebound from exhaustion and stress. Your system feels so much calmer. It treats dozens of minor ailments. Use it as a regular tea and you may never get a urinary tract infection.

Skin and Soul. In herbal lore, it's been said that the rose is good for the "skin and soul," and that can be taken literally. Rose hips tea enhances the function of everything from your skin to your innermost being. It's healing for your skin, good for your muscles and bones, tones your organs, clears mucous congestion, heals tissues, and acts on a cellular level for repair and regeneration. It fights cell damage that can be caused by free radicals. And it lifts your spirits because it's an antidepressant that gives you pizzazz!

These are the virtues of the rose:

Antidepressant	Antiviral	Urinary Tract
Aphrodisiac	Blood Tonic	Tonic

Tension Relief	Hormone	Anti-inflammatory
Nerve Strength	Regulator	Digestive Aid
Immune Strength	System Cleanser	Skin Hydration
Circulatory Aid	Stress Resistant	Phlegm Remedy
Antioxidant	Infection Fighter	Recovery Tonic
Astringent	Respiratory Aid	Adrenal Supporter
Antiseptic	Antispasmodic	Free Radical
Kidney Tonic	Antibacterial	Scavenger

Uses Through the Ages. In Chinese medicine, rose hips are called *Jing Ying Zi*, and are used for kidney energy *(Qi)* and urinary disorders. In Ayurvedic medicine, roses are mental tonics.

Beneficent Parts: Petals and hips

Properties and Values are listed above.

༃

ROSEMARY   *Rosamarinus officinalis*
The Gentle Revitalizer

There are many varieties of rosemary with different shapes and growth patterns, but when it comes to shades of blue, rosemary blooms in spectacular hues, from true blue to rosy blue, with the exception of one white-flowering variety. The official plant is a woody shrub that grows from three to six feet tall, with shiny, narrow leaves that are dark green above and soft gray below. It blooms in spring and sometimes fall with lavender-blue flowers that fill the air with a fragrance like sweet pine.

Native to the shores of the Mediterranean, France, and Spain, rosemary grows on rocky hills overlooking the sea, sending its piney perfume on the wind to sailing ships. The sheen on its leaves, damp with morning mist, led to its name *Dew of the Sea*.

A Crowning Jewel

Rosemary has enchanted poets and historians for centuries. It has a long history of medicinal use, for cooking, symbolic blessings, and aromatherapy in gardens around the world. The ancient Egyptians designed wall gardens lined with rosemary. In Algeria it was a clipped border for rose gardens. In Rome, it was a hedge around formal gardens, and in festivals, wreaths of rosemary crowned the heads of young girls and men.

The Roman armies brought it to England in the Dark Ages, and it became a prized plant in monastery gardens. When Queen Elizabeth of Hungary was paralyzed, she was massaged daily with rosemary, lavender, and myrtle, and claimed she owed her cure to rosemary.

Rosemary has always been associated with love and remembrance and prized as much as a jewel. When Anne of Cleves married England's Henry VIII, her crown was a jeweled gold coronet, intertwined with sprigs of rosemary. Brides carried rosemary in their bouquets to herald happy marriages.

Love and Remembrance. Rosemary's symbolic nature for love and remembrance are also keys to its health properties. It's a tonic tea for your heart and mind. Rosemary stimulates blood flow through your heart, which in turn enhances the supply of oxygen and nutrients to your brain. Your heart works better, and your memory and concentration are improved.

Relaxer. Rosemary may be a tonic, but it also relaxes your nervous system. This eases anxiety, depression, and tension headaches.

Recuperation. Rosemary tea is an excellent drink to take while recovering from an illness or surgery, and especially for seniors. It's an herb that gently restores immunity and health. It has antioxidants to prevent cell damage from free radicals. It relaxes and tones your nerves, enhances the flow of digestive juices, and improves your body's ability to absorb nutrients. It has no side effects, and can be taken regularly.

Scalp. Rosemary tea is a stimulating scalp rinse to activate circulation, cleanse follicles, and revitalize the area to stimulate hair growth.

Skin. Rosemary brings the blood to the skin to give you a glow, and has antiseptic value to improve your skin's ability to resist infections.

Slenderness. Rosemary improves the digestion of fats, and keeps wastes from accumulating, including cellulite deposits.

Uses Through the Ages. Rosemary has been used to fight lingering bronchial infections. Its antispasmodic properties relieve bronchial spasms to improve breathing.

Special Feature: Rosmarinic Acid

A principle ingredient in rosemary is rosmarinic acid. It's antiviral and antimicrobial to fight infections. It's also anti-inflammatory to ease inflammations.

Beneficent Part: Whole plant above the root

Properties: Volatile Oil of Rosemary, Flavonoids, Phenolic Acids, Rosmarinic Acid, Triterpenic Acids, Tannins, Bitters, Resins

Values: Antiseptic, Antioxidant, Expectorant, Decongestant, Circulatory Tonic, Digestive Tonic, Astringent, Relaxant, Carminative, Antispasmodic, Antidepressant, Diuretic

❦

SAGE   *Salvia officinalis*
Herb of Wisdom and Longevity

A Mediterranean native, sage is an aromatic brush plant with grayish-green leaves that have a soft, pebble finish. It flowers on and off through the summer with spires of purple flowers.

A Symbol of Eternal Spirit

Its Latin name *salveo* means "to heal." Throughout the ages, sage has been associated with wise men or sages. The seven branched candlestick in the Hebrew religion was inspired by the flowering spires of salvia judaica, the sage that grew in Jerusalem.

In *Virtues of British Herbs*, John Keel summed up the virtues of sage quite inspirationally:

> *Sage will . . .*
> *retard the rapid progress of decay . . .*
> *relieve that faintness, strengthen that weakness . . .*
> *prevent the hands from trembling . . .*
> *the eyes from dimness . . .*
> *and make the lamp of life, so long as*
> *nature lets it burn, burn brightly.*

The wisdom is: Sage as you age.

It was cultivated in monastery gardens, flourished in China, and was introduced to Britain in the 16th century.

In California, Spanish priests learned the secrets of sage from the Indians they were trying to convert, and sage was grown in mission gardens in El Camino Real. When Zane Gray wrote *The Riders of the Purple Sage*, he was galloping through a collection of American sages—some with silver, woody leaves and pastel flowers, or green, crinkled leaves and chocolate red flowers. Some bloom in cobalt blue, yellow, and ultramarine. American sage is considered one of the best sages, imported by the Chinese, who use sage roots to move stagnant blood and strengthen the heart.

Antiaging. Sage is antibiotic to fight infections, it's high in nutrients to tone the body, and it helps to prevent premature aging with antioxidants that keep free radicals from damaging tissues and cells.

Inspirational Tea

If you are confused about a problem that needs solving, or a tough decision you have to make, try a cup of sage tea. It has the unique ability to clear the cobwebs and bring clarity.

❧ ❧

Blood Sugar. Sage helps to lower blood sugar levels.

Digestive Remedy. Sage relaxes the muscles and soothes the lining of the digestive tract. It has bitters that ease the digestive process and increase digestive enzymes. It also calms the stomach, relieves indigestion and gas.

Liver. A stimulant for sluggish livers and associated symptoms, such as headaches, fatigue, and reduced immunity. Sage gives you vitality.

Nasal Congestion. Sage is a disinfectant, and the steam from sage tea water can be inhaled to clean your sinus passages.

Night Sweats. Sage is cooling. It can reduce sweating by almost 50 percent.

Respiratory Infections—Colds, Tonsillitis, Bronchitis, Congestion. Astringent, antiseptic, and expectorant, sage fights germs, clears phlegm, and reduces fevers. Take warm sage tea internally, and use extra tea water as a gargle to fight infections in your throat.

Sage for Women. Sage is a tonic to the reproductive system that eases menstrual irregularities. Since it reduces sweating, it can ease night sweats or "hot flashes" in menopause.

Special Features: Dandruff. Sage tea is an herbal rinse for your scalp, where it defeats dandruff. Some say that sage can restore color to gray hair.

Caution: Moderate use is best. Avoid sage if you have epilepsy.

Beneficent Parts: Leaves and root

Properties: Vitamins A, B1, B2, B3, C, Calcium, Iron, Magnesium, Manganese, Phosphorus, Potassium, Selenium, Silicon, Sodium, Sulfur, Zinc, Volatile Oil, Bitters, Tannins, Triterpenoids, Resin, Flavonoids, Estrogenic Compounds, Saponins; Root: Vitamin E

Values: Antispasmodic, Astringent, Antiseptic, Carminative, Relaxes Peripheral Blood Vessels, Reduces Sweating, Antibiotic, Lowers Blood Sugar Levels, Promotes Bile Flow; Root: Sedative, Circulatory Stimulant, Cooling

❦

SARSAPARILLA
The Deep-Cleaner

Smilax officinalis

This climbing herb of Central America has a twining stem with big prickles; large, oblong leaves with deep veins; pale flowers; and deep red berries. But it is the long orange roots of sarsaparilla that first made waves when Spanish traders brought them to Europe in the 16th century to treat syphilis. By the 18th century, sarsaparilla roots were called a cure-all.

Sarsaparilla is often called Jamaican sarsaparilla, because the first exports of its roots were from Jamaica. The word *sarsa* means "bramble," and *parilla* means "vine," signifying the herb's nature as a thorny vine.

Blood and Body Cleansing. Sarsaparilla is considered one of the best cleansing herbs for the body. It contains saponins which deep-clean the body, removing toxins through the skin (by sweating), through the urine (with its diuretic nature), from the intestines (by stimulating bowel movements), and by vacating mucous from the lungs.

Metabolism. Sarsaparilla is a metabolic stimulant, which enhances the utilization of fats, carbohydrates, proteins, and nutrients by the body.

Psoriasis, Shingles. Sarsaparilla tea can be used as a deep-cleaning skin wash to treat psoriasis, shingles, and other eruptive skin conditions.

Sexuality in Men and Women. Researchers at Pennsylvania State College found that sarsaparilla contains three hormonelike substances: testosterone, progesterone, and cortin, which affect sexuality.

1. Impotence. The natural testosteronelike substance in sarsaparilla can help to fight impotence in men who are not getting their normal supply of testosterone from the testes. It can boost the libido and bring new energy to men who are lacking testosterone.

2. Menopause. The natural progesteronelike substance in sarsaparilla can help menopausal women who lack progesterone, the hormone that tones the reproductive system and brings vitality to the libido. Recent studies suggest that the lack of progesterone at menopause may be more important than estrogen, and many women are using progesterone supplements for renewed energy in menopause. This is a decision that each woman must make individually, with the guidance of her physician.

3. Adrenal Hormone. The cortinlike substance in sarsaparilla is similar to the hormone cortin that is secreted by the adrenal glands. Without enough cortin, you can feel nervous, depressed, lacking energy, and your body can be more susceptible to infections.

Venereal Diseases. Indian sarsaparilla *(Hemidesmus Indica)* has been found to be an effective treatment for venereal diseases. (This is not the case with other sarsaparillas.)

Uses Through the Ages. Sarsaparilla was used by the

Cree Indians to treat syphilis. It has been used in Europe as an anti-inflammatory for arthritis and rheumatism. In China, it is used as a cleanser for urinary tract disorders. Sarsaparilla used to be one of the flavoring agents in root beer.

Caution: Sarsaparilla is not recommended if you have kidney or liver weakness.

Beneficent Part: Root (orange-brown roots are considered the best)

Properties: Mucilage, Saponin Glucosides, Fatty Acids, Vitamins A, B-Complex, C, D, Calcium, Copper, Good Source of Iron, Magnesium, Manganese, Phosphorus, Potassium Chloride, Silicon, Sodium, Sulfur

Values: Tonic, Blood Purifier, Body Cleanser, Alterative, Adrenal Stimulant, Diaphoretic, Deobstruent

❧

SASSAFRAS   *Sassafras officinale*
The Sweet Root Bark

A native of the United States and Canada, sweet sassafras is often used in blends for its flavor, cleansing nature, and aromatic value. It's a good tea to take for a hangover, because it quickly moves toxins out of your blood, and it's an anodyne for pain relief. It's a time-honored tea for rheumatism and gout.

Beneficent Part: Root bark

❧

SAW PALMETTO   *Serenoa serrulata*
The Libido Booster

A native of eastern North America, saw palmetto has long, slender leaves that form a fan-shaped design on the stem. Its berries are black with pale brown pulp.

Hormone Balance, Glands. Saw palmetto cleanses and strengthens glandular tissues, and helps to regulate hormone balance in both sexes.

Nervous System. Soothing to the nervous system, saw palmetto helps to relieve tension and anxiety.

Prostate, Testes, Impotence. Saw palmetto has a tonic effect on the male libido. It cleanses and nourishes male reproductive organs to prevent atrophy of the testes. It is also used to fight prostate enlargement.

Undernourished, Fatigued. Saw palmetto improves digestion and vitality, and has a long history of use as a treatment for diseases of malnourishment.

Urinary Tract Infections, Incontinence. Saw palmetto's saponin cleansers are especially good for the urinary tract to combat infections. It has been used to fight incontinence.

Women's Life Cycles. A tea for the female libido, saw palmetto helps to regulate periods, tones the reproductive tract, eases cramps and pain.

Special Feature: Fat Fighter

Saw palmetto contains the enzyme lipase that breaks down fats. It can be helpful in the treatment of obesity and overweight.

Beneficent Part: Berries

Properties: Vitamin A Carotenes, Alkaloids, Glucosides, Resins, Steroidal Saponins

Values: Antiseptic, Decongestant, Diuretic, Sedative

❧

SCHIZANDRA   *Schizandra chinensis*
The Bountiful Berries

The berries from this herb of northern China are a vitality fruit. The Chinese call schizandra *Five Taste Fruit*, because it contains all of the tastes—bitter, sweet, pungent, salty, sour. In the complex network of Chinese medicine, each taste relates to specific organs and body systems, to seats of emotions, to the five elements, five seasons, and they all interrelate to create harmony and balance. Since schizandra contains five tastes, it's good for the whole body.

Chi Tonic. In China, schizandra is called *Wu Wei Zi*, known as a vital energy tonic that is especially good for the kidneys and skin. It is used for endurance, energy, and to balance body functions. Schizandra is antibacterial to fight infections. It improves protein production and circulation, protects the liver, and tones the urinary tract. Schizandra is an *adaptogen*—an herb that has an energizing effect on human cells to help cells resist stress— physical, mental, and environmental. It is often found in blends with ginseng for vitality and youthfulness.

Libido. Schizandra is reputed to be a libido tonic for men and women.

Caution: The best way to take tonic herbs is with cautious respect. Don't start taking a tonic herb during an illness without professional guidance.

Beneficent Part: Berries

Properties: Schizandrins, Malic and Citric Acid, B-Sitosterol, Vitamins A, B-Complex, C, D, Calcium, Copper, Iodine, Iron, Magnesium, Manganese, Phosphorus, Potassium Chloride, Silicon, Sodium, Sulfur, Zinc

Values: Adaptogen, Antibacterial, Astringent, Sedative, Aphrodisiac, Kidney Tonic, Energy Tonic

❧❧

SCULLCAP
Scutellaria laterifolia
The Nerve Tonic

This Native American herb has square stems and richly textured, serrated leaves that taper at the tips. It blooms from tall, drooping spikes with blue, helmet-shaped flowers that gave scullcap the nickname *Quaker Bonnet.*

Nerves Never Had It So Good. Scullcap is one of the most respected *nervines* in the herbal kingdom. It's rich in minerals to strengthen and tone the nervous system, to help you face stress with better defenses. It is recommended for *all nervous disorders,* to alleviate tension, anxiety, the jitters, hysteria, nervous exhaustion, digestive distress, depression, panic.

Withdrawal Symptoms. Scullcap tea will ease the nervous tension and internal distress that accompanies withdrawal from alcohol, nicotine, drugs, and prescription tranquilizers. It will also help to restore your compromised nervous system. Scullcap can be found in many blends, because of its soothing qualities. Its slightly bitter taste can be perked up with honey or cinnamon.

Withdrawal Therapy Tea

Take scullcap tea in one-half cup doses, sipping it at regular intervals to maintain a steady flow of nourishment to your nerves. Repeat daily until the nervous condition is resolved, then take the tea as needed.

~∾ ∾~

Beneficent Parts: Leaves, stems, flowers

Properties: Calcium, Potassium, Magnesium, Iron, Silica, Flavonoid Glycosides, Bitter Principle, Volatile Oil, Tannins

Values: Nervine, Tonic, Antispasmodic, Mild Astringent, Digestive Aid

SENNA
A Potent Laxative

Cassia angustifolia
Cassia acutifolia

Senna is a powerful laxative and cathartic that stimulates the intestinal walls, particularly in the lower bowel. It shouldn't be used if you have an inflammatory condition, and it is best to use senna in a small amount in a blend, since soothing herbs are needed to counter the gripping effect of senna, which can be sudden, uncomfortable spasms in the intestines.

Beneficent Parts: Leaves and pods

SHEEP SORREL
The Defender

Rumex acetosella

A native of Europe and member of the buckwheat family, sheep sorrel is packed with vitamins, minerals, chlorophyll, and has carotenoids, bioflavonoids, and citric acids. These nutrients enhance the oxygen in tissues and promote new tissue growth. Sheep sorrel cleanses the kidneys, bladder, and liver, and helps to remove deposits from blood vessels, to aid the body's immune system to fight diseases of decay.

Beneficent Part: Leaves

SILYMARIN (see MILK THISTLE)

SLIPPERY ELM
Ulmus rubra
A Treasure Beyond Measure

A native of the United States and Canada, slippery elm is a grand tree that grows to sixty feet with thick gray-white bark and rough leaves with serrated edges. Its powered inner bark is cinnamon-colored, with virtues that are simply remarkable.

Barrier to Disease. Mucous membranes throughout your body are your body's natural barrier to disease. When they are infected or inflamed, resistance to disease is reduced, particularly in the organ or system where the inflammation occurs. When the inflammation remains, or the infection goes deeper, the organ or system is jeopardized, and that affects the balance of your whole body.

Slippery elm bark is one of the best restorative treatments for inflamed or irritated mucous membranes throughout your body. It draws out toxins with real fervor, and it coats the membranes with soothing mucilage to heal them, and shield them from infections.

A treatment with slippery elm can be a major step toward disease prevention. It can help to halt a disease before it escalates. It can provide stunning relief for all inflammatory conditions, including respiratory problems, lung weakness, inflammation of the stomach lining, urinary tract disorders including cystitis, and it is especially soothing for intestinal disorders, including lower bowel inflammatory disorders, colitis, and diverticulitis. It aids digestion and can normalize bowel movements with routine use. It fights acidity, and is literally a food in your system.

Disease and Recovery. Slippery elm helps to build your body's defenses to disease. Its ability to draw out toxins is superior. It soothes and protects your cells. It's a wholesome herb with as much nutrition as oatmeal, including cancer-fighting vitamins and silicon for tissue repair. It is valuable for prevention, and to give your health a boost during illness and recovery.

Nutrition Source for Building Strength. Slippery elm contains vitamins A, B-complex, C, E, K. It is high in protein, and has calcium, iron, magnesium, phosphorus, potassium, silicon, selenium, sodium, and zinc. It's ideal for recovering from any illness.

Sores, Boils, Burns, Benign Growths, Skin Diseases, and Infections. The bark powder of slippery elm is one of the best poultices to soothe inflammation, draw out impurities from the skin, speed healing, and restore the tissue's integrity. You make the poultice like a tea, but you add only a small amount of water to create a paste.

Special Feature: Protein for vegetarians and muscle builders

Recipe: Slippery elm tea can be made with warm milk or hot water. Often milk is added to a hot water tea. One-half spoonful of the bark to each cup of tea is a reasonable dose for health maintenance. You might want to take it two or three times a day for special needs.

Beneficent Part: Inner powdered bark

Properties: Powerful Nutrition, Mucilage, Starch, Tannins

Values: Health Tonic, Detoxifier, Demulcent, Emmolient, Laxative

∂℞

SMILAX (see SARSAPARILLA)

∂℞

SPEARMINT
The Flavoring Mint

Mentha spicata
Mentha viridis

Known as *garden mint*, spearmint is the herb that is often mistaken for peppermint because it pops up in gar-

dens and has a minty scent. Both mints have similar
properties, but peppermint's volatile oil of menthol is not
equaled in quality by any other kin in the mint family,
and that sets them apart.

Spearmint is a Mediterranean mint with lance-shaped
leaves and spikes of purple flowers. Since it resembles
peppermint, but is not as costly to cultivate, spearmint is
the mint that is frequently used in blends for flavoring
and synergy. It's soothing to your nerves, excellent for
motion sickness and to stop hiccoughs. It may not be the
elite mint, but it made up for that by being the friendly
mint in chewing gums, good for sore throats and to
freshen the breath. It's often used to clear sinuses, to
regulate acid/alkaline balance, and for urinary tract distress. It has also been used to cleanse and tone the
spleen.

Beneficent Part: Whole Plant

❧

ST. JOHN'S WORT   *Hypericum perforatum*
The Restorer

A native of Britain, Europe, and Asia, St. John's wort
is a wild perennial that grows along roadsides, in meadows, and in woody places. It has a wispy appearance with
straight stems and small pale green oblong leaves. It
blooms from June to August with delicate bright yellow
flowers. The flower petals and leaves are dotted with oil
glands that produce a red resin or volatile oil. After
blooming, it produces small black seeds that have a res-
inous scent.

Its name *hypericum* translates from Greek as "over an
apparition." According to myth, St. John's wort was so
offensive to evil spirits that one whiff of the aroma forced
them to flee.

Two saints are credited with giving St. John's wort its name. One was St. John of Jerusalem, who used the wort (plant) during the crusades to heal his knights' battlefield wounds, and the other was John the Baptist. One legend claims that the plant grew from the blood of John the Baptist when he was beheaded, and the red oil from its glands represents his blood.

The 16th-century physician Paracelsus extolled the virtues of St. John's wort as surpassing all other medicinal herbs when he wrote: ". . . In all formulas, there is no medicament that is so good and without detriment, without hazard, as the healer St. Johnswort . . . its virtue shames all formulas . . ."

Antidepressant and Restorative Nerve Tonic. St. John's wort is one of the finest *nervines* in the herbal kingdom to restore the nervous system after prolonged periods of exhaustion and stress. When it is taken as a routine tea, it can lift depression, anxiety, and irritability, stabilize the emotions, and ease insomnia. It contains hypericin, which is an MAO inhibitor and stimulant for dopamine, which eases depression. The tea is cooling and bittersweet.

Immunity. Research from New York University and the Weizman Institute of Science in Israel found that hypericin and pseudo-hypericin, two of St. John's wort's properties, inhibited growth of the HIV virus in animals. Current studies are underway with a synthetic version of hypericin to test the effect in humans. St. John's wort is also high in flavonoids; it's antiviral, antibacterial, and antifungal to fight disease.

Incontinence. St. John's wort has been used to treat incontinence, the tea taken before bed.

Menses, Menopause. St. John's wort has a sedative effect to relieve pain and discomfort in menses, tension, and depression in menopause.

Neuralgia, Neuritis. St. John's wort relaxes the muscles, reduces inflammation, and eases pains in the nerves for neuralgia and neuritis.

Strains, Sprains. A warm tea bag of St. John's wort can be a compress to relieve localized nerve pains and inflammation in strains and sprains, including tennis elbow.

Uses Through the Ages. St. John's wort has been a treatment for bladder disorders, lung disorders, and jaundice. It also has a reputation as an external application to dispel hard tumors.

Caution: Regular use can make you sun-sensitive. Avoid during radiation therapy since it can heighten the tendency of the skin to blister or redden. St. John's wort can increase blood pressure, cause headaches and nausea in some individuals. It should not be used in combination with prescription drugs, including MAO inhibitors, steroid medications, tranquilizers, or over-the-counter diet pills or amphetaminelike drugs. Short-term use is best.

Beneficent Parts: Plant and flowers

Properties: Good Source of Flavonoids, Glycosides, Rutin, Tannins, Volatile Oils, Resins

Values: Astringent, Analgesic, Anti-inflammatory, Sedative, Tonic for Nervous System

⌘

STRAWBERRY, WILD   *Fragaria vesca*
The "Cool" Citrus Herb

A member of the rose family and a northern hemisphere native, wild strawberry is often called *Alpine Strawberry* for its home in the Alps. It has light green leaves with deep seams and scalloped edges, and it produces a delicate cone-shaped scarlet berry dotted with tiny brown seeds. The leaves and berries are often separated for teas, so check your box of tea to see if it contains the leaves or dried berries.

Leaves: A tea of wild strawberry leaves is excellent for your overall health, soothing for gastrointestinal inflammations and infections, digestive disorders, and rheumatic gout. Because of their "cooling" nature, wild strawberry leaves are often used to balance other herbs in blends.

Berries: A whole body tonic, tea from the berries of wild strawberry is valued as a recuperation tonic after illness or surgery. The berries are a good source of iron and vitamins to nourish the blood, strengthen the body, and cleanse the liver of "heat" toxins, which makes the tea especially useful for recovery from hepatitis.

Special Feature: Eczema

The berries of wild strawberry are good for the skin, and are recommended as a remedy for eczema. The tea used in a bath can help to take the redness from a sunburn.

Beneficent Parts: Leaves and berries

Properties: Citric Acids, Mucilage, Volatile Oil, Pectin, Sugar, Vitamins B, C, E, Salicylates, Minerals

Values: Astringent, Liver Tonic, Cleanser, Diuretic (Mild), Laxative, Heals Burns, Wounds

❧

SUMA   *Pfuffia Paniculata*
The Vitality Root   *Martius Kuntze*

A member of the Amaranth family, this Amazon native can reach eighteen feet in the wilds. Some species have stunning flowers that resemble dangling tassels in deep purple-red.

The Greek translation of *Amaranth* means "unfading," or "not to die away," and the term was often used by poets who dreamed of a flower that never died. Suma is an herb that is used for unfading energy and long life. In Spanish, it is called *Para Todo*—"for all things."

Cellular Oxygenation and Immunity. Cells need oxygen to retain their health. Suma is unique for cellular integrity. It has a high concentration of the antioxidant germanium, which protects cells from free radical damage that can accelerate aging and cellular decay. It also contains beta-ecdysone, an enzyme that works with germanium to oxygenate cells. It has antitumor saponins, and stimulates the production of interferon for immune strength. It's a good tea to take for chronic immune weakness.

Energy and Endurance. Suma has been called *Brazilian ginseng*, because it is a vital energy tonic, but its nature is quite different from ginseng. Suma's energy is gentle and deep, and it doesn't contain the testosteronelike properties of many ginsengs, which can lead to a wired-up feeling, particularly in women. Suma was used by the Xingu tribe for three centuries as a vital energy tonic and purifier. It increases energy, endurance, and alertness, but it does it in a mellow way, because of its aphrodisiac qualities. It has nineteen amino acids and allantoin, which helps to build muscle. It has vegetable hormones that lower blood cholesterol and improve circulation. It's an *adaptogen*—an herb that balances opposites. It's an excellent tea for menopause, chronic fatigue, to restore vital energy. Suma has a plain taste, and you might want to use it in a blend, or charm it with a spritz of orange.

Beneficent Part: Root

Properties: Germanium, Amino Acids, Vitamins A, E, K, Some Bs, Minerals, Iron, Zinc, Silica, Magnesium, Cobalt, Vegetable Hormones, Allantoin

Values: Vital Energy Tonic, Adaptogen, Purifier, Aphrodisiac

❧

TANG KUEI (see DONG QUAI)

❧

THYME   *Thymus vulgares*
The Knockout Infection Fighter

This European native flourishes in Mediterranean regions, and can be found in Spain, Asia Minor, Algeria, and Tunis. It's a low-growing shrub from the mint family with tiny gray-green leaves, whorls of pink flowers, and an invigorating balsam scent.

There are two versions for the origin of its name. In Greek, *thyme* means "to fumigate," and the Greeks burned the herb as a disinfectant. Also from the Greek, *thumus* means "courage"—the attribute that is historically linked with thyme. In medieval England, knights were given scarves from their ladies, embroidered with a sprig of thyme and a bee, to signify courage and bravery.

Bronchial Dilator. Thyme tea can be a valuable health treatment to strengthen your respiratory tract, and fight infections that may be lingering there. It opens your bronchial tubes for cleansing, expectorates phlegm, and it's a decongestant for your chest. Its powerful antiseptic action cleanses your respiratory tract of fungal, bacterial, microbial, and viral infections. It clears your head, throat, windpipe, bronchial tubes, and lungs. Begin by taking a mild tea once a day for a week, then gauge your progress. As you begin to feel less tightness in the chest, you can use the tea less frequently.

Infections—Colds, Flu, Viral. A cup of thyme tea can be the tonic you need to make a real breakthrough with an infection, septic condition, or to aid your recovery from disease. It's the most powerful antiseptic herb—antiviral, antifungal, antimicrobial, and antibiotic. There aren't many germs that can withstand that kind of clout. You can also use thyme to clean sickroom air by boiling the herb in an uncovered pot on your stove, letting thyme's antiseptic steam purify the air.

Skin Infections. Thyme tea is a four-star antiseptic for all skin infections, including parasitic skin problems and those that resist synthetic antibiotic treatment. When it is applied topically, thyme increases the blood flow to the area and purges the infection. Soak a cotton ball with thyme tea and press the liquid into areas on your skin that need cleansing and healing. Even if your infection is deep-seated, stay with the antiseptic wash until the condition is healed. Thyme is also used as a wash to kill ringworm.

Urinary Tract and Kidney Infections. If there's an unhealthy invader causing an infection in your urinary tract, thyme tea will wipe it out, even after other methods have failed. Its antiseptic action is particularly valuable to cleanse your kidneys.

Uterine Disorders. Thyme was called *Mother Thyme* for its motherly treatment of uterine problems.

Special Feature: Local Fungal Infections

Thyme tea can be used to treat a fungal infection on-site.

Athlete's Foot. Restore your feet with an antifungal foot soak. Prepare a potent cup of thyme tea with two tea bags (or two teaspoons of dried herbs). Add the warm tea to a bucket of water. Use a deep bucket to insure that the water covers your ankles to treat hardened ankle areas. Repeat until the condition is resolved.

Fingernail Fungus. Restore damaged nails by soaking your hands in thyme tea water, made from one tea bag (or one teaspoon of dried herbs). This is a useful monthly treatment for people who have routine manicures to prevent infections.

Mouth and Throat. Use thyme tea as a throat and mouth gargle to conquer fungal infections in the mouth, including thrush.

Nasal Cleanse. To fight infections, polyps, growths, and fungal allergies, use one thyme tea bag (or one spoonful of dried herbs) in a pot of boiling water as a steam inhalant for your sinuses.

Beneficent Parts: Leaves, flowers, stems

Properties: Volatile Oil with Thymol Antiseptic, Flavonoids, Tannins, High in Chromium and Manganese, Vitamins B-Complex, C, D

Values: Antiseptic, Antibacterial, Antibiotic, Antifungal, Antimicrobial, Antispasmodic, Aromatic, Astringent, Broncho-dilator, Carminative, Decongestant, Diaphoretic, Expectorant, Emmenagogue, Tonic, Expels Worms

৯৫

UVA URSI   *Arctostaphylos uva-ursi*
Also called BEARBERRY
A Bear of an Astringent

At home in hilly regions, uva ursi can be found in the mountains of Europe, Asia, America, and the hills of Scotland and Ireland. It's a small shrub with light brown bark, trailing stems, and shiny evergreen leaves. It blooms with waxlike flowers in close clusters that are white and red, and it produces a vivid red berry.

Urinary Tract Infections. Uva ursi's unique ingredient is arbutin, a tranquilizer and diuretic that is broken down in your system to an antiseptic which cleans your urinary tract as it is being excreted. It is also valuable to cleanse excess uric acid from your system. It is astringent and soothing, used for inflammations and infections in the urinary tract, including cystitis in women and urethritis in men.

Uses Through the Ages. Uva ursi dates back to the 13th century, when it was used by Welsh physicians. It has been used as a tea for bladder, kidney, and uterine disorders, and to cleanse the pancreas and spleen.

Special Feature: Contains allantoin, which promotes new cell growth
Beneficent Part: Leaves

Properties: Arbutin, Allantoin, Gallic Acid, Ellagic Acid, Tannins, Vitamins A, B-Complex, B3, C, Calcium, Iron, Magnesium, Manganese, Phosphorus, Potassium, Selenium, Silica, Sodium, Zinc

Values: Nutrient Tonic, Antiseptic, Astringent, Diuretic

✍

VALERIAN   *Valeriana officinalis*
Nature's Tranquiliser

This native of Europe and Asia likes temperate climates and marshy areas by woods and rivers. It has dark green, segmented leaves, and one long stem that rises from the root and can reach five feet in height. There are 150 species of valerian, including Japanese valerian—*Kesso Root*, one called *Pretty Betsy*, another called *Drunken Sailor*, and American valerian—*Lady Slipper* or *Nerve Root*, but the official plant is identified by its small pink-tinted white flower clusters.

The yellowish root has an interesting arrangement of strands that look like tangled nerves—the specific problem that valerian treats.

Phu Phu

Valerian has an odd aroma when it is blooming, and this gave it the name of *Phu*. Its name comes from the Greek *valere*, which means "to be in health."

The Thompson Indians of British Columbia carried valerian in their medicine bags to apply to wounds.

In World War I in England, valerian was given for air-raid strain, and proved to be an effective weapon against nerve damage.

Tranquilizer and Sleep Aid. Sedative to the higher nerve centers, valerian relieves pain, tension, and the effects of excessive strain to bring sleep in stressful situations, with no morning-after effects. It quiets and soothes the brain and nervous system. It should not be taken along with sleep-inducing medications, since it will enhance their effect. Low doses are recommended, and regular breaks (every two or three weeks) are suggested. It's best to use valerian in small amounts in blends.

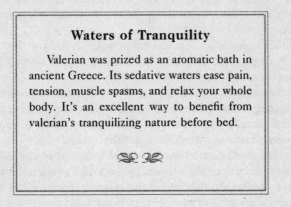

Waters of Tranquility

Valerian was prized as an aromatic bath in ancient Greece. Its sedative waters ease pain, tension, muscle spasms, and relax your whole body. It's an excellent way to benefit from valerian's tranquilizing nature before bed.

Vision. Valerian has been used to strengthen the eyesight, particularly if the weakness is in the optic nerve.

Uses Through the Ages. Valerian has been used for hysteria and stress-induced nervous disorders.

Caution: Use very moderately. A small percentage of users (5 percent) can have hallucinatory reactions to valerian.

Beneficent Part: Root

Properties: Good Source of Niacin, Calcium, Vitamins, and Minerals; Volatile Oil—Isovalerianic Acid, Valepotriates, Alkaloids, Iridoids

Values: Tranquilizer, Antispasmodic, Expectorant, Diuretic, Carminative, Mild Anodyne

✦

VERVAIN   *Verbena officinalis*
Also called BLUE VERVAIN
The Nerve Tonic

Native to Europe, China, and Japan, vervain is a bright green perennial found in pastures and by roadsides. It has lance-shaped leaves that are deeply lobed and rough to the touch. The leaves form opposites on a long stem and bloom along the top with tiny white flowers.

Vervain's legend is second to none. It grew in Jerusalem, and is said to be the herb that was used to stop the bleeding and heal the wounds of Jesus.

It's known as *The Herb of Grace*, and for centuries in Europe, it was a sacred herb, blessed before harvest, and used for religious rituals. Its official name comes from the Roman *verbena*, which means "alter-plant."

The herbalist Pliny, in A.D. 77, said that the Magi claimed that people who are rubbed with vervain "obtain their wishes, banish fever, and cure all diseases." It was once worn around the neck to bring good luck.

Aphrodisiac. Vervain has aphrodisiac properties to ease anxiety, depression, lethargy, headaches, and irritability.

Nerves. Vervain is sedative and tonic to the nervous system. It calms you down and strengthens your ability to withstand stress.

Gums (Spongy). Use vervain tea as a mouthwash.

Uses Through the Ages. Vervain has been used for fevers, excess uric acid conditions, and to ease the pain of neuralgia, sprains, bruises, and wounds.

Caution: Avoid vervain if you have bronchial conditions or asthma, since it can be a bronchial constrictor. Its best use is in moderate amounts in blends.

Vervain Nightcap

Vervain's sedative and aphrodisiac nature make it a good nightcap to strengthen your nerves while you sleep.

Beneficent Part: Whole plant, picked before flowering

Properties: Vitamins C, E, Calcium, Manganese, Citrol-Volatile Oil, Bitter Glycosides-Iridoids, Tannins

Values: Nervine, Sedative, Antispasmodic, Liver Tonic, Laxative, Bile and Uterine Stimulant

VITEX (see CHASTE BERRY)

WHITE OAK   *Quercus alba*
The Antiseptic Bark

A powerful astringent and antiseptic for internal cleansing, white oak bark is good for the thyroid, liver, spleen, gums, veins, and capillaries. Because of its potent cleansing nature, white oak bark is often found in remedies for infections, particularly in the reproductive tract, including yeast infections and sexually transmitted diseases, such as herpes. It's reputed to prevent hair loss. Small amounts in blends is the recommended dose.

Beneficent Part: Bark

❧

WHITE WILLOW   *Salix alba*
An Anti-inflammatory

This native of central and southern Europe is a tower-ing tree with gray bark; slim, spearlike leaves; and drop-ping spikes of yellow flowers without petals, called catkins.

Inflammation. White willow bark has anti-inflam-matory "salicylic acid" and is often found in blends for neuralgia, arthritis, rheumatism, bursitis, and lumbago. It can also be useful for inflammatory skin conditions, since it reduces the inflammation and has nutrients for skin healing, which include vitamins A, C, and zinc.

Uses Through the Ages. White willow bark has been used to treat dyspepsia, to strengthen the digestive or-gans, and for recovery from debilitating diseases. It has also been a remedy for chronic diarrhea and dysentery.

Beneficent Part: Bark

Properties: Vitamins A, B-Complex, C, Calcium, Phosphorus, Mag-nesium, Manganese, Potassium, Salicylic Acid, Selenium, Sodium, Tan-nins, Zinc

Values: Tonic, Astringent, Antiseptic, Anti-inflammatory, Rids Worms

❧

WILD YAM   *Dioscorea villosa*
The Progesterone Root

There are more than 150 varieties of wild yam, and many are used as food. Wild yam is relaxing to the mus-cles, soothing to the nerves, and good for the glands. It's a source of vitamins and minerals, including vitamins A, B-complex, calcium, magnesium, and zinc. The Chinese variety is considered a long-life herb. One of the unique features in the Mexican variety of wild yam is its natural plant progesterone, which can be converted to corticosteroids by the adrenal glands. This has focused attention on wild yam as an herb for menopausal women, since the plant hormones may help to prevent osteoporosis. Wild yam is recommended as a tea for arthritis and irritable bowel syndrome.

Beneficent Part: Root

≫

WOOD BETONY
Stachys officinalis

The Herb of Sanctity

Growing wild in shady woods, wood betony has tall, hairy stems; rough, fringed leaves; and pink to purple flowers with white spots that bloom in whorls from short spikes. A characteristic that is unique to wood betony is its interrupted spike—there is a break in the flower rings—a bare stem followed by more flowers.

Held to High Standards

Highly regarded in the Middle Ages, wood betony was also called *Bishopswort*, cultivated in monastery gardens and churchyards, and often worn as a necklace to keep perils away and sanctify the wearer. Even animals were purported to know the benefits of wood betony, and one tale tells that stags pierced by arrows would search for wood betony to eat for their cure.

According to an old Italian proverb, it was better to sell your coat than go without betony. And in Spain, to praise someone they would say he had as many virtues as betony. Augustus Caesar's physician recorded dozens of diseases that betony could cure. In 9th century Saxony, it was said that betony was good for the head and soul, could shield a man from bad visions and dreams, and banish despair.

Herbs that are *alteratives* like wood betony work their charm very subtly, bringing healthy changes with calming sensations.

Head Clearing. Wood betony's name comes from the Celtic *betonica*, which means "good for the head." It was once the foremost remedy for all ailments of the head and brain. It's a circulatory tonic that is especially attuned to brain function, where it calms the nerves and clears the channels to soothe and revitalize overactive minds. Techniques that are used to relieve stress, such as yoga or meditation, often refer to centering as "coming down out of your head." Wood betony tea has a similar head-clearing effect. It relieves congestion, and eases a "heavy head"—an aching feeling in the bones in back of your head and face that can often hang on after a cold or sinus condition.

Digestive Disorders. Wood betony is a gentle digestive remedy to soothe indigestion, heartburn, dyspepsia, colic, and gas.

Headaches. Poor circulation to the brain, tension, and a sluggish liver are often linked with headaches. A cup of wood betony tea relieves all three, since it is a circulatory tonic, liver enhancer, and relaxing. In old England, it was taken as powdered snuff for headaches.

High Blood Sugar Levels. The alkaloid trigonelline in wood betony lowers blood sugar levels.

Neuralgia, Sciatica, Arthritis, Gout, Rheumatism. Wood betony tea can bring relief from pain and tension. It's excellent for your nervous system, and you derive many other benefits. It's one of the herbs that works on many levels to make you feel better all over.

Skin Infections, Varicose Veins. Wood betony's tannins are astringent to stop bleeding, repair cuts and wounds, and fight infection. The warm tea in a soft cloth can be a comforting compress for skin infections, cuts, sores, and varicose veins. You will be surprised at how quickly it starts to heal and seal. The water also penetrates the skin to provide deeper healing.

Beneficent Part: Flowering Plant

Properties: High in Calcium; Also Has Magnesium, Manganese, Phosphorus, Potassium—Tannins, Saponins, Alkaloids

Values: Circulatory Stimulant Attuned to the Brain, Digestive Stimulant, Nerve Tonic, Wound Healer, Astringent, Liver Cleanser

∾

YARROW
Achillea millefolium
The Wound Healer

Yarrow is a hardy perennial with a noble history and a weedy persistence to grow anywhere—in fields, pastures, meadows, and even dry barrows by the roadside.

It has small, feathery leaves; rough stems; and thin, white silky hairs that cover the entire plant. The term *millefolium* translates as "thousand leafed," and in olden days, yarrow was called *Milfoil* or *Thousand Leaf*. From June to September, yarrow blooms with clusters of miniature flowers in delicate hues that range from sweet lilacs, soft reds, rosy pinks, whites, or hot yellow, according to the variety.

Yarrow in Battle

Yarrow's legend and the derivation of its name *Achillea* dates back to the Trojan War. It's the herb that the warrior Achilles used on the wounds of his soldiers to stop bleeding and speed healing. Through the ages, yarrow traveled with the military as a *vulnerary*—wound healer. Since one method of delivering an herb's vital properties to the system is by absorption through the skin, Achilles' soldiers were being treated to yarrow's other healing benefits as well.

Blood Purifier. Yarrow gets your circulation going to clear out toxins, and fight bacteria in the blood.

Digestive System. Yarrow tea is a well-rounded treatment for digestive difficulties. It fights inflammations and infections in the stomach lining and intestines. It has bitters that tone the digestive tract, and it relaxes internal spasms.

Fevered Colds. As a tea for those "killer" colds with high fevers, yarrow is an aggressive warrior. It removes body heat to break a fever, fights infections, reduces mucous, and relieves congestion.

Sweat That Cold

The old adage about sweating a cold is real with yarrow tea. It hunts down toxins fast and sweats them out of your body, leaving you cool, decongested, and a bit giddy. Drink plenty of water afterward.

❧ ❧

Menstruation. Yarrow has been used to regulate menstrual cycles, reduce heavy bleeding during periods, and ease uterine congestion.

Oh Sweet Melancholy! Yarrow is known to chase away the blues by clearing out toxins and toning the liver. In olden days, it was taken as *Milfoil tea*, and it's still used today to treat liver deficiencies.

Veins (Varicose, Hemorrhoids). Yarrow is anti-inflammatory, to shrink swollen veins, and antiseptic to heal them. Drink your tea, but don't discard the tea bag. Break open the bag, use the warm herb as a poultice on a varicose vein, and cover it with a Band-Aid to fight the problem from both sides. For hemorrhoids, try a yarrow sitz bath.

Wounds. In ancient times, yarrow was called *Herbe Militaris* ("The Military Herb") and *Soldier's Wound Wort*. It has the warrior's seal of approval to clean and heal cuts, burns, ulcers, and inflamed skin conditions. It has silica to repair damaged tissues. Wash wounds externally with cooled yarrow tea water, or soak a bandage in yarrow tea to cover the wound.

Uses Through the Ages. It's been used to reduce high blood pressure, calm an irritable bladder, and soothe painful joints. In Norway, fresh yarrow is eaten as a cure for rheumatism. In Sweden, yarrow is called *Field Hops*, used to make beer, since it's more intoxicating than hops.

Special Feature: Fighting Hair Loss

Some say yarrow prevents baldness if it's used as a scalp wash. You can use yarrow tea as a scalp rinse to invigorate your scalp, remove toxins, and stimulate the area. It's best for dark-haired people.

Beneficent Part: The whole plant, gathered in August, fully flowered

Properties: Vitamins A, B-Complex, C, E, Bioflavonoids, Choline, Iron, Inositol, Magnesium, Phosphorus, Potassium, Selenium, Silicon, Sodium, Volatile Oil, Coumarins, Lactones, Amino Acids, Sterols, Bitters, Flavonoids, Tannins, Saponins, Salicylic Acid, Sugars, Cyanidin

Values: Astringent, Vulnerary, Anti-inflammatory, Antiseptic, Digestive Tonic, Antispasmodic, Diaphoretic, Hypotensive, Diuretic

❧

YELLOW DOCK   *Rumex crispus*
The "Cool" Cleanser

A member of a wild family of docks, yellow dock is often found in roadside ditches and dry areas. It has long, lance-shaped leaves that rise straight from the root and curl at their edges. The flower stem also rises from the root, with smaller, alternating leaves, and tiny, delicate flowers that spring from the base of the upper leaves. The most striking feature of yellow dock is underground—the bright orange root looks like a carrot.

Anemia. There's iron in that root to build red blood and combat fatigue.

Laxative/Cleanser (Fast Acting). Yellow dock has a similar laxative effect to rhubarb, but there's no discomfort or pain.

Acid Balance. It reduces acidity, soothes the stomach and bowel lining.

Psoriasis, Eczema. Yellow dock's common use is for inflammatory skin conditions, and blood-related skin diseases. It detoxifies tissues, breaks congestion, and reduces inflammation to facilitate healing. Take as a cool tea.

Lymph Congestion. Yellow dock removes toxins, reduces inflammation and lymph buildup, and takes the wastes from the body ASAP.

Skin Itching. A yellow dock tea bath takes the *itch* out of itchy skin.

Fibroids. Yellow dock has been used to control uterine fibroids, and ease menstrual irregularities such as heavy bleeding.

Uses Through the Ages. Yellow dock's cleansing properties make it useful for bowel infections, peptic ulcers, arthritis, and rheumatism.

Caution: Yellow dock has oxalic acid which can be an irritant in high doses.

Beneficent Part: Root

Properties: Good Source of Iron; Has Vitamins A, B-Complex, and Minerals, Glycosides, Tannins

Values: Cooler, Cleanser, Laxative, Increases Bile Flow, Astringent, Diuretic, Liver Tonic

❧

YERBA MATE
Ilex paraguayensis
Also called MATE
The High-Energy Tonic

A member of the holly evergreen family, this South American shrub is found in Brazil, Argentina, and Paraguay, often in the wilds, growing to twenty feet. It has large green leaves with serrated edges, white flowers, and red fruit. It's also known as *Paraguay Tea*, and is considered the national drink of Argentina.

Its name comes from *yerba*, for "excellence," and *mate*, to refer to the *matti gourd* which was traditionally used to hold the brew. Native Indian ceremonies with mate tea were social and spiritual occasions, where guests were invited to share the gourd of tea, which was often spiced with burnt sugar and lemon juice, and drunk through a straw (usually silver), with a bulb strainer at the end to filter the bulk from the water.

Energy. Yerba mate is a physical and mental energy tonic. It provides vital nutrients to the brain, to improve memory and concentration. It delays lactic acid buildup in strenuous exercise, and improves motor responses. It contains pantothenic acid, which boosts metabolism, to help the body utilize carbohydrates, fats, proteins, and vitamins, and break down cholesterol, steroids, and fatty acids.

Mate Celebration

Have mate the native way. Sauté brown
sugar with lemon juice, brown it in the pan,
and add it to your yerba mate tea. Mmmmm!

❧❧ ❧❧

Fatigue. Fights fatigue with balanced nutrients.

Nervous System. Tonic and nutrient source for sound
nerves.

Sexual Energy. Yerba mate is a stimulant for the adrenal cortex, which is a regulator of androgenic hormones. Some say mate is a sex tonic, and that's not
surprising, since it has considerable nutritive value. It
might seem more energizing to men, but both sexes take
it.

Spine. Tonic for spine and nerves.

Stress. Yerba mate builds resistance to stress. It contains B vitamins and C—the antistress team. Pantothenic
acid (B5) stimulates the adrenal glands, which regulate
production of hormones, including adrenaline and cortisone.

Uses Through the Ages. Yerba mate has been used
for energy, and as a sustaining source of nutrition. Often,
the only food that natives carried when they went on
long journeys was the yerba mate leaves for tea.

Beneficent Part: Leaves

Properties: Vitamins A, B-complex, B1, B2, B3, B5, C, E, Biotin,
Choline, Inositol, Calcium, Hydrochloric Acid, Iron, Magnesium, Manganese, Phosphoric Acid, Potassium, Silica, Sodium, Sulphur, Chlorophyll, Fiber, Resins, Volatile Oil, Tannins, Xanthine, Mateine, Bitters,
Trace Minerals

Values: Stimulant, Diuretic, Aperient, Laxative, Astringent, Purgative, Fever Reducer, Rejuvenator

৵৯

YERBA SANTA
Eriodictyon glutinosum
The Bronchial Balm

A native of California and New Mexico, yerba santa is an evergreen shrub with smooth stems that are coated with sticky resin. It has smooth yellow-toned leaves that are thick and leathery with a deep middle seam, and it blooms with blue flowers in clusters.

It has been called *Holy Herb,* and *Consumptive's Weed* for its beneficial effect on the bronchial passages, larynx, and lungs. It clears congestion and phlegm, and makes saliva flow.

Uses Through the Ages. American Indians rolled and smoked the dried leaves for asthma. It is used in California as an expectorant. Yerba santa is often found in blends for asthmatic conditions.

Beneficent Part: Leaves

Properties: Five Phenolic Compounds, Glycerides of Fatty Acids, Volatile Oil, Resin, Glucose, Phytosterols

Values: Digestive Stimulant, Tonic, Expectorant, Aromatic

References

Barney, Paul D., M.D., "The Cranberry Cure," *Herbs for Health*, Nov/Dec 1996.

Blumenthal, Busse, Goldberg, Gruenwald, Hall, Klein, Riggins, and Rister, *The Complete German Commission E Monographs, Therapeutic Guide to Herbal Medicines*, Austin, TX: American Botanical Council, 1998.

Brooks, Svevo, Ed., *The Protocol Journal of Botanical Medicine*, Ayer, MA: Herbal Research Publications.

Burton Goldberg Group, *Alternative Medicine, The Definitive Guide*, Fife, WA: Future Medicine Publishing, Inc.

Byler, Emma, *Plain and Happy Living, Amish Recipes and Remedies*, Cleveland: Goosefoot Acres Press.

Chevallier, Andrew, *The Encyclopedia of Medicinal Plants*, New York: DK Publishing Inc.

Dunne, Lavon J., *Nutrition Almanac*, Third Edition, New York: McGraw-Hill.

Farwell, Edith Foster, *A Book of Herbs*, Piermont, NY: The White Pine Press, Inc.

Foley, Daniel J., *Herbs for Use and Delight, Selections from the Herbarist*, New York: The Herb Society of America, Dover Publications, Inc.

Foster, Steven, "Fighting Depression the Herbal Way," *Herbs for Health*, Nov/Dec 1996.

Foster, Steven, "Herbs for Health," *The Herb Companion*, Dec/Jan 1995/1996, Loveland, CO: Interweave Press, Inc.

Greenwald, John, "Herbal Healing," *Time*, Nov. 23, 1998, www.time.com.

Grieve, M., F.R.H.S.; Leyel, C.F., ed. *A Modern Herbal*, New York: Hufner Press, Div. of Macmillan Publishing Co., Inc.

HerbalGram, American Botanical Council, P.O. Box 201660, Austin, TX 78720–1660.

Hill, Madalene; Barclay, Gwen, "Vanilla," *The Herb Companion*, Dec 1995/Jan 1996.

Hobbs, Christopher, *Ginkgo, Elixir of Youth*, Santa Cruz, CA: Botanica Press.

Hobbs, Christopher, *Handbook for Herbal Healing*, Santa Cruz, CA: Botanica Press.

Howe, Maggy, "The Chinese Medicine Chest," *Country Living*, September 1996.

Hudson, J. L., Seedsman, *The Ethnobotanical Catalog of Seeds*, La Honda, CA.

Jarvis, D. C., M.D., *Folk Medicine*, New York: Ballantine Books, Div. of Random House, Inc.

Jones, Kenneth, "Pau d'Arco," *Herbs for Health*, Nov/Dec 1996.

Kamen, Betty, Ph.D., *Hormone Replacement Therapy, Yes or No*, Novato, CA: Nutrition Encounter.

Kuts-Cheraux, A. W., B.S., M.D., N.D., *Naturae Medicina and Naturopathic Dispensatory*, Yellow Springs, OH: American Naturopathic Physicians and Surgeons Association, Antioch Press.

Lowe, Carl, "Natural Mood Boosters," *Energy Times*, Nov/Dec 1997.

Marion, Joseph B., *Anti-Aging Manual, The Encyclopedia of Natural Health*, Woodstock, CT: Information Pioneers.

McIntyre, Anne, *The Complete Woman's Herbal*, New York: Henry Holt.

Mindell, Earl, R.Ph., Ph.D., *Herb Bible*, New York: Simon and Schuster/Fireside.

Morton, M. S., et. al., "Lignans and Isoflavonoids in Plasma and Prostatic Fluid in Men: Samples From Portugal, Hong Kong, and the United Kingdom," *Prostate*, 1997.

Mowrey, Daniel, Ph.D., *Herbal Tonics and Therapies*, Avenel, N.J.: Wings Books/Div. of Random House.

Mowrey, D. B.; Clayson, D. E., "Motion Sickness, Ginger and Psychophysics," *Lancet*, March 1982.

Murray, Michael, N.D., "Cimicifuga Extract (Black Cohosh): A Natural Alternative to Estrogen for Menopause," *Health Counselor*, Vol. 8, No. 2. Green Bay, WI.

Murray, Michael, *Natural Alternatives to Over-the-Counter and Prescription Drugs*, New York: William Morrow, 1994.

Ody, Penelope, *The Complete Medicinal Herbal*, New York: Dorling Kindersley, Inc.

Quimme, Peter, *Coffee and Tea*, New York: New American Library.

Rector-Page, Linda G., N.D., Ph.D., *Healthy Healing*, Sonora, CA: Healthy Healing Publications.

Reid, Daniel, *The Tao of Health, Sex and Longevity*, New York: Simon & Schuster Inc.

Rose, Jeanne, *Modern Herbal*, New York: Perigee Books.

Schardt, David, "Herbs for the Nerves," *Nutrition Action Health Letter*, Vol. 25, No. 8, Center for Science in the Public Interest, Washington, D.C.

Swedish Herbal Institute, Ltd., *"Clinical Summary Chisandra-Adaptogen and Schisandra Chinensis,"* York Harbor, ME.

Thompson, L. U., et. al. "Flaxseed and Its Lignan and Oil Components Reduce Mammary Tumor Growth at a Late Stage of Carcinogenesis," *Carcinogenesis*, 1996.

Tye, Larry, "Herbal Renewal," *The Boston Globe Magazine*, July 13, 1997.

Tyler, V.E., *Herbs of Choice, The Therapeutic Use of Phytomedicinals*, New York: Hayworth Press.

Wallace, Edward C., N.D., D.C., "Arthritis Pain Relief," *Energy Times*, February 1998.

Weil, Andrew, M.D., *Spontaneous Healing*, New York: Alfred A. Knopf, Inc.

Weinberger, Stanley, C.M.T., *Candida Albicans: The Quiet Epidemic*, Larkspur, CA: Healing Within Products.

Wren, R. C., F.L.S., *Potter's New Cyclopaedia of Botanical Drugs and Preparations*, New York: Pitman Publishing Corporation.

Wright, Jonathan V., M.D., "Hormone Replacement Therapy, Weighing the Risks," *Great Life*, March 1998.

Resources

❧

If you have difficulty finding herbs as boxed teas or dried herbs for teas in your area, the following toll-free numbers will give you a jump-start to get teas in boxes or dried herbs for teas. These resources will mail anywhere in the United States.

Teas in boxes (as ready-to-use tea bags or in bulk)
Country Health, 1–888–640–5757. Ask for tea department.

Loose dried herbs by the ounce
Purple Shutter Herbs, 1–888–865–HERB

The author's correspondence
P.O. Box 6243
Holliston, MA 01746

The American Botanical Council
Herbal Gram is a publication of the American Botanical Council, which gives you current updates on herbs and excellent information. Write the American Botanical Council, P.O. Box 201660, Austin, TX 78720–1660 for information.

Index

❧

Victoria Zak is an award-winning writer, researcher, and co-author of *The Fat to Muscle Diet* and *The Dieter's Dictionary and Problem Solver*. Her work has appeared in many national publications, including *Ladies' Home Journal, Prevention, Shape, USA Today, The Boston Globe,* and *Glamour*. She lives in Massachusetts and has been featured in *Who's Who in the East*.